Interpersonal Wellness System

Improving Your Interpersonal Intelligence

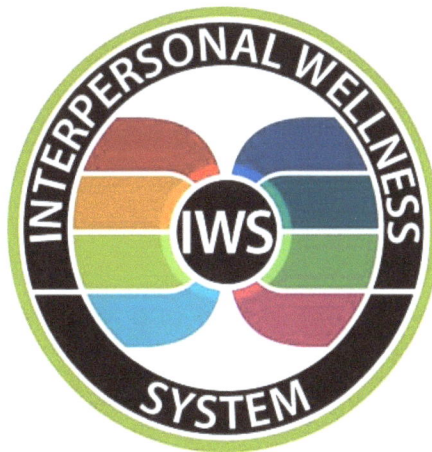

A Coaching Tool Kit

Interpersonal Wellness Services Inc.

Helping You Improve Interpersonal Intelligence

ACKNOWLEDGEMENTS

A Time to Experience Your Best Self

Thank you for showing interest in the Interpersonal Wellness concept and this workbook. I applaud your efforts to take action in creating the life or workplace experience you desire. I know that you will find the Interpersonal Wellness Quotient (IWQ) concept informative, enlightening, revealing and transforming.

As a coach, I know the value of acknowledgement and would like to thank some of the individuals who have been instrumental in my vision for this work and who have contributed to the completion of this workbook.

A special thanks to my brilliant daughter Dellorn, for your vigour and tenacity for life and for helping to work on this project. You inspire me. To my dear aunts, especially Ann Albert, for her encouragement and kind words, and to my growing network of certified Interpersonal Wellness Coaches - I have learned a lot from you; please don't stop giving to the world. I also want to acknowledge my many clients who have contributed to my learning over the years.

My gratitude also goes to my husband Misan and to my son Misan Jr. for quietly being there and tolerating my absent-mindedness.

Special thanks to my team of skilled Associates and friends who have contributed feedback in the development of this workbook.

Note on source material: This workbook draws on excellent resources and my many experiences working with organizations and clients in Pre-mediation coaching and Interpersonal Wellness Coaching (IWC). The names and roles in this workbook are fictitious and do not mirror entirely any one person's experience, but are a combination of situations and responses that I have addressed over the years.

Interpersonal Wellness Quotient (IWQ) ® is a Registered Trademark

Interpersonal Wellness System (IWS) ® is a Registered Trademark

© 2010, Joyce Odidison
Interpersonal Wellness Services Inc.
13 - 875 Gateway Rd
Winnipeg, MB, Canada. R2K 3L1
204.668.5283 Phone
204.667.8845 Fax
877.999.9591 Toll-Free
E-mail: admin@interpersonalwellness.com
Web: www.interpersonalwellness.com

Interpersonal Wellness Publishing, 2010

Printed and bound in Canada by Art Bookbindery
www.ArtBookbindery.com
ISBN 978-0-9736067-1-3

Content

A Time to Reconnect

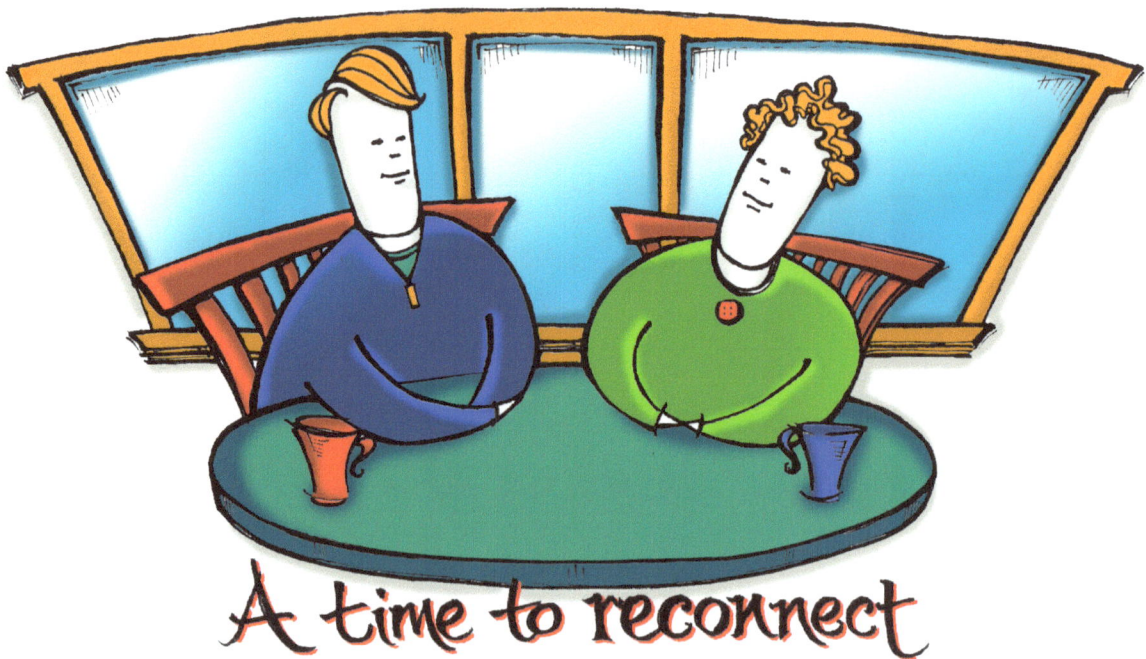

Introduction

If you are distressed by anything external, the pain is not due to the thing itself, but to your estimate of it; and this you have the power to revoke at any moment.
    -Marcus Aurelius Antoninus

Introduction

What if you lived your life as if every thought, action or choice had a consequence on how you experienced your relationships? What if you believed yourself to be a system of interconnected parts that ultimately affected each other? Would you be more deliberate in your thoughts and actions?

I believe that when we fully grasp this concept, our world will become a much better place to live. Only then will we engage each other in healthy interactions and learn to successfully negotiate our life and work relationships. Consequently, we will make fewer mistakes with special relationships and take corrective actions to put things right when a challenge occurs.

What if you believed that every thought you held had a physiological impact on you? Would you be more deliberate about what thoughts you held onto and which ones you let go? I believe this is true and I'm convinced that it is our responsibility to guard our minds from destructive thoughts that may lead to actions and patterns that are unhealthy and destructive to our life success.

Ask yourself, how often have you repeated the same self-defeating patterns or find yourself committing to unproductive and unhealthy habits? Could these be as a result to a certain pattern of thoughts you hold? This book is designed as a tool kit that will allow you to go deeper within your thoughts and explore the deeply held beliefs that has encumbered you. Through this process you will access a roadmap for developing new thoughts that will improve your life relationships.

We each have the capacity to contribute to life in either a positive or negative way. When we go through life unaware of this fact, we become unconscious contributors, who create situations and outcomes we do not like. No one chooses to go through life with a blindfold but many of us do just that. To be intelligent is to be clever, aware and knowledgeable.

Intelligent people know what they have to offer and how to use it for their success. They also know how to go about finding the information they need to show off their brilliance. In this book, I want to engage you in removing the blindfolds that you may have been wearing and replace it with 20/20 vision. I intend to stimulate your thoughts and share a bold concept that will allow you to think differently about your life and your relationships.

If you are tired of the infighting, and bickering and want to reduce the incidents of broken relationships, miscommunication, divorces, conflicts, broken homes and displacement of people, then read on. I intend to help you find a way to contribute to a reality in which people work well together and know how to negotiate and communicate their feelings appropriately.

This book is based on the concept of the Interpersonal Wellness System (IWS) model and on the measurement of one's system, aptly named the Interpersonal Wellness Quotient (IWQ). This measurement will help you determine how well you are doing in all areas of your life, revealing how much you are able to contribute to the wellness of your relationships. Let's face it; we can only give from what we have. We either have enough to give or we need to get more so that we can give more. Measuring your IWQ will reveal whether you have enough to give or need to top up your wellness factor in any given area. One's IWQ can range from low to high. Those who are experiencing difficulties in their relationships may want to examine their own ability to contribute to their relationships, by measuring their IWQ to learn where they can make improvements that may benefit their relationships and improve their life success.

This simple but revealing IWQ assessment will shift your awareness and concept of yourself in relationships and show you how to reduce some of the relationship challenges that you face. You will become aware of yourself as part of a larger system that is connected by vibrations, atmosphere and energy. Alerting you to your ability to create and impact yours and others wellness, and your ability to change these vibrations.

It is easy to become consumed with our work and our careers, family needs and other life challenges. In so doing, we become isolated, disengaged, removed and disconnected from those around us. It is very easy to see ourselves as removed from and apart, as observers of what is going on around us. The truth is that we are all connected, and when we become aware of ourselves, our choices, actions and their consequences on us and those around us, we are able to unleash the best of ourselves to their benefit. What a beautiful experience!

I have the pleasure of seeing my clients reach new heights of personal discovery and growth using the IWS model and the IWQ assessment. This is continually surprising and thrilling. I have therefore come to believe that we never truly reach perfection in this lifetime. Our journey here is about identifying continuous growth opportunities, allowing us to gradually change, develop grow and become our better self.

Measuring your capacity to contribute to your work or life relationship is an empowering and enlightening experience. This allows you to see where you are doing well in your life. I encourage you to take time to celebrate your life successes and all the areas where you are doing well. When you encounter an area where you have not devoted the required time for growth and development, I encourage you to acknowledge the lack, and begin thinking of who you can become with future growth. If you don't like what is revealed, you hold the power to change your results, so take steps to change it.

If we don't know how much money we have in the bank, we have a high likelihood of over spending. In the same way, it is important for us to know our IWQ, because this tells us how much we are able to contribute to our relationships and life's other demands. Once we know what we have to offer, we can make intelligent choices about how to engage and with whom.

Not knowing is an excuse we no longer have. We are all aware of the sufferings and misery that have been caused by embittered interactions in our lives and communities. We see far too many relationships fail or end poorly because those involved lack the ability to contribute meaningfully to their relationships.

There are too many divorces, broken homes and broken hearts in our world. We know of people who have developed high stress levels, chronic illnesses and diseases because they have over committed or over taxed their system. Not knowing what you are able to contribute to life and your relationships can be deadly. I would like to provide everyone with a tool to quickly and easily scan and assess their wellness and their capacity to contribute well to their life and relationships.

It is no secret that we all have an area in our lives that need some improvement. If left unmonitored, a lack of growth in this area can manifest as poor interpersonal skills and become a problem for those in our network of relationships. It may show up as bad attitude or even poor social skills. This book will provide you with a quick and easy way to do your own self assessment. I encourage you to use this workbook to assess, grow and develop any or all dimensions of your life and exceed even your own expectations.

Foundation

Interpersonal wellness is a reality in all our lives. Everything we do has a consequence to ourselves and to others. Whether we want to or not we affect those around us with our negative or positive attitudes and interactions.

 After many years of responding to negative interpersonal conflicts, researching, writing and teaching about pre-mediation, coaching and interpersonal conflict management, I developed the Interpersonal Wellness System® model and the Interpersonal Wellness Quotient® (IWQ) metric and coaching to help my clients get faster and more consistent results.

The IWQ metric is a measurement of all the dimensions of one's wellness system. The foundation of the IWS model is that we are each a system of interconnected, multidimensional parts that require continual assessment, and growth to help us grow and become extraordinary human beings with the potential to live exceptional lives.

As you go through this workbook, I encourage you to be open minded and focus on your ability to develop and maintain the kind of relationships you want, in order to create the kind of life you desire. Nothing is impossible. I have worked with individuals who have had very divisive, conflicting relationships and by applying some of the strategies in this tool kit they now have much happier and respectful relationships.

As your level of interpersonal intelligence increases, you will develop new ways to solve problems, and to discern potential challenges. You will also become more confident in yourself, your skills and abilities, enough to risk taking steps to address challenging situations effectively.

By measuring your IWQ you will become aware of your capacity to contribute to a work, business or personal relationship well. The model emphasizes that you need to know what you are able to contribute, by insisting that those who manage the wellness of all areas of their lives will have great lives and healthier relationships, while those don't will end up creating intolerable situations for themselves and others.

We commonly witness friends, relatives and colleagues suffer burnout because they are giving more to a relationship, to work or life than they have the capacity to. This is equivalent to buying a Mercedes when you can only afford payments on a Suzuki. It is your job to be intelligent about managing your life relationships. After working through this book you will have a higher level of awareness of what you can contribute and you will be better equipped to negotiate life more successfully.

When you are low in gas it is your responsibility to stop and fill up, but if you drove your car with a broken gas gauge you wouldn't be able to tell how empty or full your tank was and you could end up running out of gas and stranded on an isolated stretch of highway. By measuring your IWQ, you will know your capacity to contribute and be able to make intelligent decisions about your life and relationships.

To do this, you will conduct an assessment of your life that will reveal your IWQ, which is a measurement of your wellness in all eight dimensions of your life, to determine how well you are doing in these areas. By looking at the Interpersonal Wellness System model on the next page, you will notice what goes on in each dimension will ultimately impact each other and overall what you have to contribute to your life and relationships.

There is no exception to this rule, and when we learn this fact and take more deliberate actions, we will find ourselves living the kind of lives we want to live. No one is exempted from this life reality. If you have a belly button, then you have an IWQ. You just don't call it that or are unaware of it. If it's the latter, this means that you are not in control of your life and that is not the plan.

Take Control of Your Life!

Measuring your IWQ puts you in the driver's seat of your life by providing you with information to make the decisions necessary for the success of your life relationships. If you are unhappy with your relationships, you should begin by asking questions of yourself first. This will help you to assess and determine how much you are contributing to the wellness of your relationships. Only then can you approach the other person and ask them what they are willing to do to contribute to the wellness of the relationship.

For every failed relationship there is a pattern of behaviour that contributed to its demise. It is unfortunate that those in the relationship failed to see the signs and patterns, or they felt powerless to change things at the time.

By assessing and calculating your wellness in any five areas in each dimension of the IWS model and dividing the sum of your scores by eight, you will be able to discover your IWQ. This will give you a handle on what you might do differently and help you assess your capacity to contribute to healthy interactions in your work or life relationships – your interpersonal network.

Jack's Story

Jack is in his early forties and a father of three. He is newly divorced and is trying to make sense of his life. He has a lot of debts, finds himself in awkward social situations, makes poor judgments in his intimate relationships, is having conflict with his teenagers, ex-wife and neighbor, and is now having problems at work with his new boss.

Jack's friend told him about life coaching and he contacted the Life Coaching Centre and began working with one of the coaches. One of the first exercises Jack completed with his coach was the Interpersonal Wellness Quotient (IWQ). From this assessment, Jack wanted to gain more awareness of what was happening in each dimension of his life, so he identified five areas in each dimension that was relevant to his current life situation as a an employed, single divorced dad and ex-husband.

From this exercise, Jack wanted to become aware of the thoughts he held that motivated his actions and led to the negative consequences he was experiencing. He also hoped to find a way to change some of the patterns he had developed and set goals to take control of his life. He believed that if he could only become aware of those thoughts and change his thinking and consequently his actions in time, he would become the CEO of his own life and have more control of his actions and ultimately change his results.

Interpersonal Wellness System Model

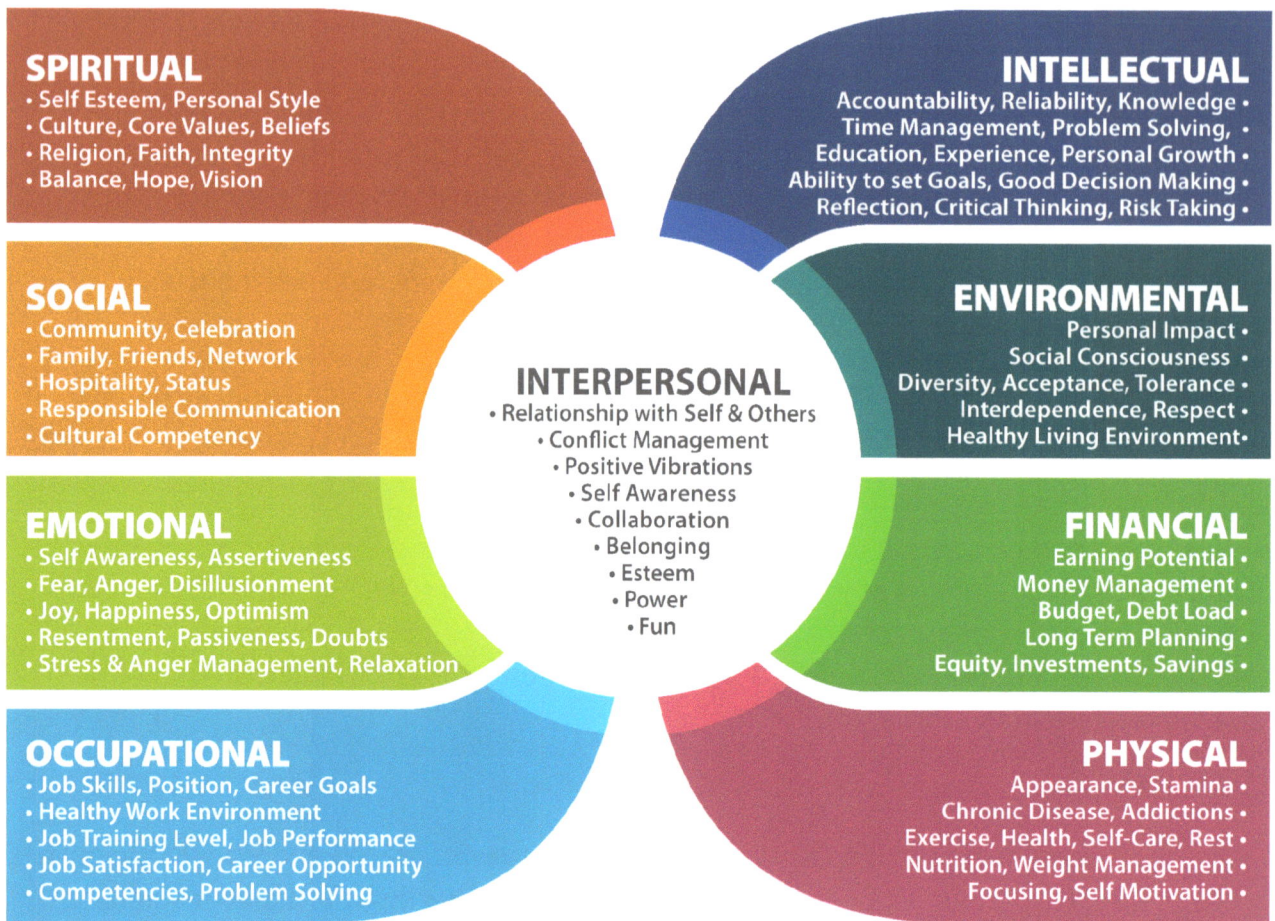

SPIRITUAL
- Self Esteem, Personal Style
- Culture, Core Values, Beliefs
- Religion, Faith, Integrity
- Balance, Hope, Vision

SOCIAL
- Community, Celebration
- Family, Friends, Network
- Hospitality, Status
- Responsible Communication
- Cultural Competency

EMOTIONAL
- Self Awareness, Assertiveness
- Fear, Anger, Disillusionment
- Joy, Happiness, Optimism
- Resentment, Passiveness, Doubts
- Stress & Anger Management, Relaxation

OCCUPATIONAL
- Job Skills, Position, Career Goals
- Healthy Work Environment
- Job Training Level, Job Performance
- Job Satisfaction, Career Opportunity
- Competencies, Problem Solving

INTERPERSONAL
- Relationship with Self & Others
- Conflict Management
- Positive Vibrations
- Self Awareness
- Collaboration
- Belonging
- Esteem
- Power
- Fun

INTELLECTUAL
- Accountability, Reliability, Knowledge
- Time Management, Problem Solving,
- Education, Experience, Personal Growth
- Ability to set Goals, Good Decision Making
- Reflection, Critical Thinking, Risk Taking

ENVIRONMENTAL
- Personal Impact
- Social Consciousness
- Diversity, Acceptance, Tolerance
- Interdependence, Respect
- Healthy Living Environment

FINANCIAL
- Earning Potential
- Money Management
- Budget, Debt Load
- Long Term Planning
- Equity, Investments, Savings

PHYSICAL
- Appearance, Stamina
- Chronic Disease, Addictions
- Exercise, Health, Self-Care, Rest
- Nutrition, Weight Management
- Focusing, Self Motivation

® Joyce Odidison

Here is how Jack assessed his IWQ. He rated himself in five areas in each of the eight dimensions that were important to him, based on a scale of 1 to 10, where 10 is excellent and 1 is poor. He gave himself a number based on how well he thought he was doing in that area between 1 and 10. Then he added all five numbers in each dimension then divided this total score by 5, resulting in a score of 3.8, for example, in Spiritual wellness.

This means that he has the capacity to give a possible 3.8 out of a possible 10 in the area of spiritual wellness to his life and work relationships. He did the same scoring for the other 8 dimension in the IWS model with the following results: Social: 5, Emotional: 4.2, Occupational: 5, Intellectual: 4.8, Environmental: 4, Financial: 2.6 and Physical: 7.2. He then added these scores to a sum of 36.6, which he divided by 8 to get his IWQ: 4.75.

This exercise can be very enlightening and helps you come to grips with your capacity to contribute to your interpersonal network. It can also motivate you to take steps to attain an IWQ that is satisfactory and fulfilling.

Spiritual	Social	Emotional	Occupational	Intellectual	Environmental	Financial	Physical
Self-esteem: 2	Community: 5	Self-awareness: 5	Job Skills: 7	Accountability: 3	Diversity: 4	Earning Potential: 4	Appearance: 8
Values: 4	Family: 5	Fear: 4	Position: 4	Knowledge: 5	Social Consciousness: 4	Money Management: 4	Stamina: 6
Balance: 2	Personal Growth: 4	Anger: 4	Career Goals: 4	Education: 5	Personal Impact: 4	Debt Load: 2	Exercise: 8
Trust: 2	Responsible Communication: 4	Disappoint-ment: 4	Job Satisfaction: 5	Experience: 5	Awareness of Self: 5	Budget: 3	Rest: 9
Personal-style: 6	Family: 7	Regrets: 4	Career - 5	Cognitive Skills: 6	Awareness of Others: 3	Planning: 2	Nutrition: 5
Total =16	Total = 25	Total = 21	Total = 25	Total = 24	Total = 20	Total = 13	Total = 36
Total ÷ 5 = 3.8	Total ÷ 5 = 5	Total ÷ 5 = 4.2	Total ÷ 5 = 5	Total ÷ 5 = 4.8	Total ÷ 5 = 4	Total ÷ 5 = 2.6	Total ÷ 5 = 7.2

<u>Total sum of 8 dimensions ÷ 8= Jack's IWQ = 4.75</u>

From the IWQ assessment, Jack became armed with the necessary information to make changes in his life. He began working with his coach to improve all the areas above in his life where he scored less than 5 points. This led to Jack improving his relationship with his ex-wife, resulting in a huge change in his teenagers' choices due to their ability to co-parent collaboratively. He was also able to sit down with his new boss to develop a list of areas where he needed to improve his performance and worked with his coach to do so. He is also now best buddies with his neighbour and he has a relationship with someone who has the same life goals as he does.

When he completed his exit IWQ assessment three months after coaching, Jack had an IWQ score of 7.2. He told his coach that he now feels like the CEO of his life and is no longer feeling like a victim. Jack also made dramatic improvements in his financial and his physical wellness. He lost 15lbs and was making timely payment on his newly consolidated loan. You too can have the success Jack had in his life by measuring your IWQ.

A healthy level of personal wellness is important for success in life. We cannot take our ability to interact well with others for granted. In our homes, workplaces and communities, interpersonal wellness is a measure of healthy relationships that results in joint contribution by all persons involved. It is the responsibility of all members of the group, family or workplace to maintain a healthy level of interpersonal wellness. This way it will be easy to repair infractions and remedy slights and oversights. When parties fail to maintain a healthy IWQ, everything becomes an issue and small infractions are then escalated to entrenched conflicts and disputes.

I encourage you to embrace this opportunity to reflect on your own personal development as you work on your own or with a coach. Having a coach will help you gain results faster and easier but you can also do the work on your own if you feel up to the task. This is your own special time to create whatever you desire in your life.

When you use the IWS model in the following section to measure your IWQ, be prepared for a revealing view of how you contribute to the wellness of your relationships, and plan to develop new skills and competencies so you can reach your desired IWQ. Remember, now that you are wiser about your reality it is your responsibility to make a difference and begin to live the life that you want.

Later in the book as you embark on improving your IWQ, you may find yourself challenged to take a different route, take new risks, or make changes in your attitude, actions or vocabulary that may be uncomfortable and unfamiliar. Like anything else in life worth having, a change in your IWQ will come from taking risks. Don't give up on yourself. Just keep moving ahead and you will find that it will become easier as time pass.

Remember, intelligent people know what they have to offer and how to use it to their best advantage. As you improve your IWQ, you will also be improving your level of interpersonal intelligence and the opportunity to realize more of life successes.

Questions

How comfortable are you with risk-taking?

What concerns or fears do you have about personal change?

When was the last time that you were acknowledged for something you did well?

Notes

_____

_____

When life knocks you down, try to land on your back, because if you can look up, you can get up! Let your reason get you back up.

— Les Brown

A Time to Explore

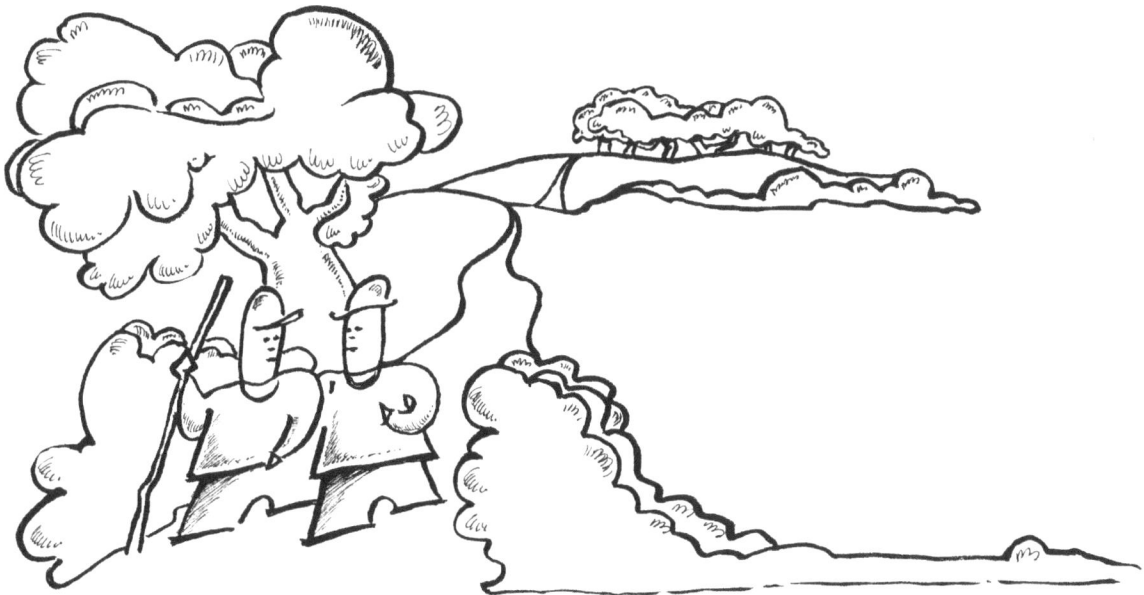

Interpersonal Intelligence

Your time is limited, so don't waste it living someone else's life. Don't be trapped by dogmas-which are living with the results of other people's thinking. Don't let the noise of others' opinions drown out your own inner voice; and most important, have the courage to follow your heart and intuition. They somehow already know what you truly want to become. Everything else is secondary.

- Steve Jobs

Interpersonal Intelligence

Interpersonal intelligence is realized when those interacting are knowledgeable of their capacity to impact their relationships in a manner that is productive. It is when they act positively in this knowledge and their actions fulfill the desired outcome of the collective. You are probably reading this workbook in hopes of improving your IWQ, which will in turn increase how intelligently you execute your life and experience your relationships. Your quest may be stemming from personal dissatisfaction, or a request from someone you work or live with to change, or to improve your interpersonal interactions.

Whether you are working to improve relationships in your personal or work life, it is imperative that you see yourself as having control.

All organizations want employees with great interpersonal skills and who relate well to others. An individual may have the highest credentials and outstanding capabilities, but if they lack essential interpersonal skills, these stellar qualities will be overshadowed.

In order to receive optimal placement, retention and promotion, **strong Interpersonal Wellness skills are essential! Those with high IWQ will ultimately have greater relationship success.**

You Create Your Reality

If you are unhappy with your current IWQ, it is most likely not all the fault of the other person(s) in your relationship. Doing your Personal Wellness Audit (PWA) in each of the eight dimensions will help you assess where you are and what you want to do differently in your life. As you reflect on your score in each dimension, think of where you want it to be in three to six months.

Questions

What current reality in your life are you aware of creating?

_____

_____

Is there something in your life that you unconsciously created?

_____

_____

Now that you are aware of your creative ability, what will you do differently in your life?

_____

_____

A Framework for Interpersonal Wellness

Those who experience optimal wellness in their life radiate positive social vibrations. They have a positive impact on those around them and foster great relationships. Conversely, those who fail to keep themselves well tend to radiate negative social vibrations to those around them, fuelling strife and conflicts.

The IWS model will help you identify the gap between your desired life and your current reality. It is my hope that you will be open to closing this gap. Too often we sit in impotence believing that we cannot change our circumstances now, nor can we take actions to change our future. Our society has programmed us to have a victim mentality. We are not victims; we each have an amazing capacity to create our own life relationships by the choices we make every day.

Religious book such as the Bible, Torah, Koran and others teaches that there is an element of faith and work necessary for creating change. This means that it takes human effort and divine intervention for successful outcomes to be reached. Your effort may be in the form of learning a new skill, changing old habits, moving past a hurt or gaining a new perspective.

As you work through the following chapters of this book, ask yourself: what skill(s) do I need to learn to improve my wellness in this area?

Because we live such busy lives we seldom take time to assess all eight dimensions of our lives and the multiple areas that each represents. Not surprisingly, new research is alerting social scientists to the fact that those who have essential life skills to negotiate and manage their lives have less stress, resulting in fewer bouts of illnesses and chronic diseases, including depression and cardiac disease, even in cases where they are hereditary.

As I write this book, new research from the University of Calgary, AB in Canada has revealed that pet owners who are caring for ill pets experience a dramatic improvement in their own health. They saw that diabetics who had pets such as dogs or cats with diabetes were much more successful caring for their own diabetes and were living much healthier lives. The cause social scientists revealed, was that they were making more conscious choices about diet and exercise for their pets and for themselves. Another example of how deliberate we can be in our actions when we have the right motivators to stimulate our awareness.

Questions

What new skill(s) do you think you will need to develop to get through this book?

_____

What could be a motivator for changing an area of your life?

_____

_____

The Interpersonal Wellness System

The IWS model views each person as a system of several interconnected parts (dimensions), whether we manage them well or not. We are born into a family, live in a community or work with a group, and by default, this comprises our interpersonal network.

We can make choices on whether to broaden, change or reduce our socializing in this network, but we are inherently social beings.

The Interpersonal Wellness System (IWS) model shows that whatever happens in one area of your life will impact the others.

The Concept

According to the IWS model, the individual is a system of eight interconnected dimensions. The activities and wellness of each affects the others, and can impact one's entire wellness system and ultimately, one's interpersonal relationships.

A challenging situation in any area will pull resources from one or more of the other areas to compensate. However, if continued over a long time, the compensating areas will become tapped out and this will result in a major drain on the resources of the other dimensions and the entire system will become taxed.

For instance, if left unattended, poor family relationships in the social dimension will affect the emotional, spiritual, physical, occupational, environmental and financial areas. If left unresolved, this will eventually impact one's entire interpersonal network; and negatively affect their self-esteem (the way one perceives self) in social groups, such as family or work relationships.

It is recommended therefore that each dimension be developed with supporting structures in place to maintain the wellness of that dimension. This practice will become very beneficial and result in reducing the need for overcompensation in any one area.

Questions

Are you experiencing a long-term stress or challenge in any area of your life? If so, for how long?

_____

_____

Is there a time when you felt you had control of this situation? If so, when and what did you do differently?

_____

_____

As you review the IWS model in the introductory chapter, is any one dimension demanding your attention?

_____

_____

Social Vibrations

Social vibrations can be referred to as the energy or atmosphere one generates. We each impact our surroundings by the thoughts we think and the attitude we display. This is a direct result of how we manage our wellness in each dimension of our life. If we manage our wellness we will send out positive vibrations, which will have positive consequences on our interpersonal relationships.

When we are experiencing wellness in all eight dimensions of our lives, we send out positive social vibrations to those around us. However, if we are unwell, the reverse happens. In order to improve wellness and create synergy, one must do a Personal Wellness audit to identify areas requiring development and growth.

This will ensure that you make a positive contribution to your interpersonal network through the improvement of your own wellness or skills. Remember, you can only give what you have, and like it or not, we are all connected and impacted by each other's social vibrations. The energy we send out to those around us can be either negative or positive. We often don't have a way to describe it except to say things don't feel good or that group morale is low. The IWQ metric will provide new language for us to describe this and to score this phenomenon. This will be beneficial for creating our new or different reality.

Questions

Assuming we communicate through social vibrations, what vibrations might you be sending out in your interpersonal network? (Rate yourself on a scale of 1 to 10, 10 being high and 1 being low.)

___ Anger
___ Fear
___ Pessimism
___ Cooperation
___ Negative Thoughts
___ Assertiveness
___ Aggressiveness
___ Passiveness
___ Contentment
___ Vulnerability
___ Doubt
___ Resentments

___ Disillusionment
___ Optimism
___ Negative thoughts

Would you need to work with a coach to change any of the above?

_____

_____

Where have you experienced negative social vibrations?

_____

_____

_____

Is there a time when your social vibration is positive?

_____

_____

_____

Taking Action

Now that you are aware of your IWQ and your need for further growth and development, you can take the necessary actions to make that happen.

There are times when the necessary change is so extensive that we need support or to work with someone else to reach our goals and there are times when we can do it on our own. As you assess your wellness in all eight dimensions, you can decide if you need to work with a coach or can do it on your own.

Whatever your choice, the most important factor is that you are taking action towards achieving the IWQ you desires.

Questions

Would you describe yourself as an action-taker?

_____

Do you have any preferences with working on your own or with a coach?

_____

_____

What is one action you have already taken since beginning this workbook?

_____

_____

Self -Direction

The goal of the IWS model and tools is to help you to become more self-aware and to help you to notice your actions and consequences and become more self-correcting. This means that you will become aware enough to correct your behaviour before you act in a manner that you don't like. I also hope that you will also become more self-directive. This means that will become skilled in schooling your thoughts and action towards continuing to grow into your best self.

Questions:

What might you gain by becoming more self-aware?

_____

_____

_____

If you were to become more self-correcting, how would your actions change?

_____

_____

_____

If you were to become more self-directing, how do you imagine this would impact your interpersonal relationships?

_____

_____

_____

Interpersonal Wellness Audit

So few of us take time to live well, we rush through life with busy schedules and seldom take time to reflect on our behaviours and their impact on others. Sometimes we get so busy we fail to acknowledge a bad habit or attitude in a particular area of our life.

IWQ is structured around you and your realities. It will provide you with a visual framework within which to audit your Personal Wellness in each of the eight life dimensions.

Questions

Do you find yourself rushing through life?

_____

_____

What are some things you may have failed to acknowledge, or let drag on?

_____

_____

Is there an area of your life where you want to devote more time?

_____

_____

A wellness audit will measure your success in all the eight dimensions of the IWS model. I hope that this will raise your awareness and help you to connect more fully with self and others.

The audit is meant to help you assess your IWQ. It puts you in touch with your core values, personal beliefs and personal style.

Measure and Know Your IWQ

Do Jack in the introduction section of this book and how he scored his IWQ, well now it's your time to get some of the awesome results that Jack experienced.

I think that everyone deserves and opportunity to change. No matter your circumstances, what you have done or where you are now. Even if you think your relationship is beyond help, this exercise will help you begin identify where you can make small steps in your life that will impact your future life relationships.

Now I would like to give you the opportunity to measure your IWQ.

Please review the IWS model on the next page and assess any five categories in each area to give yourself a score on a scale of 1 to 10 (where 10 is excellent and 1 is poor). Remember this measures poor to excellent, not high and low. Add your five scores and ÷ it by 5 to get your wellness in each dimension. Then your IWQ is determined by adding your scores in all 8 dimensions and then ÷ if by 8.

Interpersonal Wellness System Model

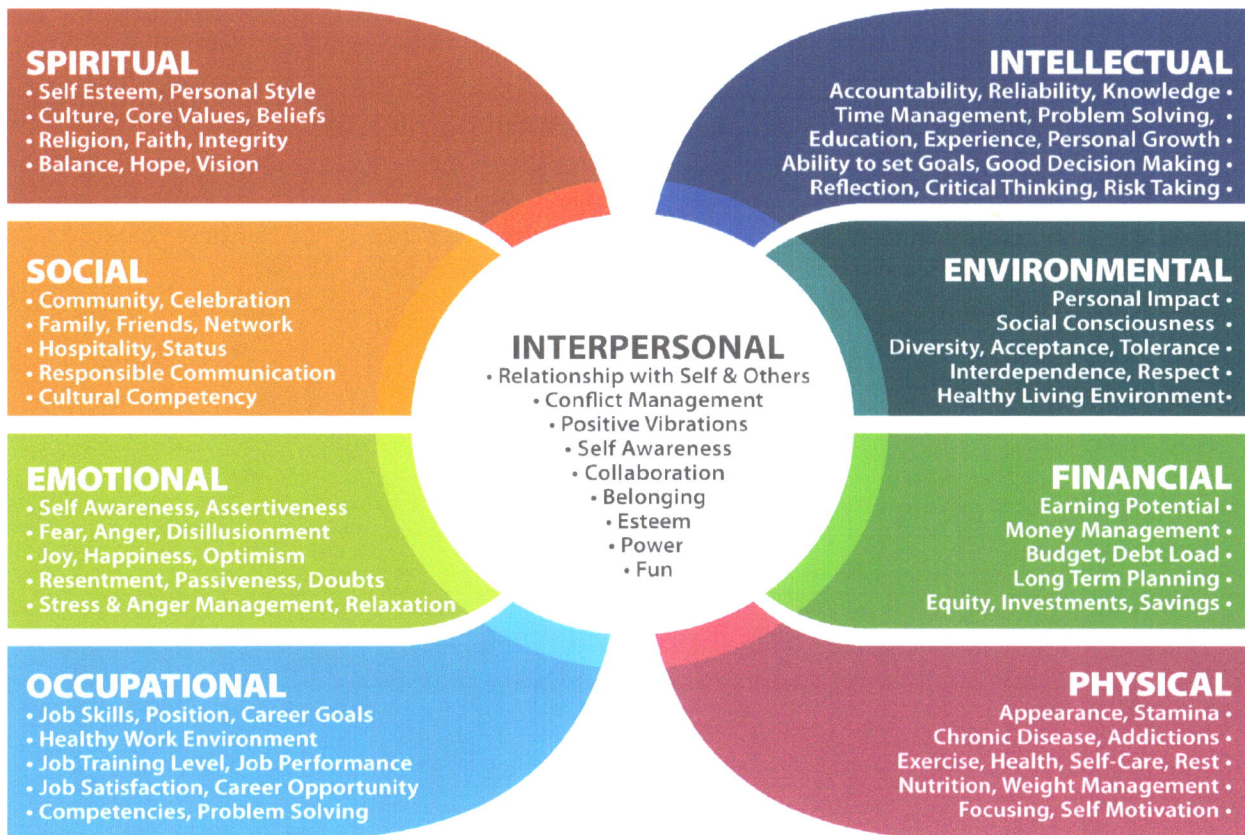

SPIRITUAL
- Self Esteem, Personal Style
- Culture, Core Values, Beliefs
- Religion, Faith, Integrity
- Balance, Hope, Vision

SOCIAL
- Community, Celebration
- Family, Friends, Network
- Hospitality, Status
- Responsible Communication
- Cultural Competency

EMOTIONAL
- Self Awareness, Assertiveness
- Fear, Anger, Disillusionment
- Joy, Happiness, Optimism
- Resentment, Passiveness, Doubts
- Stress & Anger Management, Relaxation

OCCUPATIONAL
- Job Skills, Position, Career Goals
- Healthy Work Environment
- Job Training Level, Job Performance
- Job Satisfaction, Career Opportunity
- Competencies, Problem Solving

INTERPERSONAL
- Relationship with Self & Others
- Conflict Management
- Positive Vibrations
- Self Awareness
- Collaboration
- Belonging
- Esteem
- Power
- Fun

INTELLECTUAL
- Accountability, Reliability, Knowledge
- Time Management, Problem Solving,
- Education, Experience, Personal Growth
- Ability to set Goals, Good Decision Making
- Reflection, Critical Thinking, Risk Taking

ENVIRONMENTAL
- Personal Impact
- Social Consciousness
- Diversity, Acceptance, Tolerance
- Interdependence, Respect
- Healthy Living Environment

FINANCIAL
- Earning Potential
- Money Management
- Budget, Debt Load
- Long Term Planning
- Equity, Investments, Savings

PHYSICAL
- Appearance, Stamina
- Chronic Disease, Addictions
- Exercise, Health, Self-Care, Rest
- Nutrition, Weight Management
- Focusing, Self Motivation

® Joyce Odidison

Interpersonal Wellness Quotient (IWQ)

Spiritual	Social	Emotional	Occupational	Intellectual	Environmental	Financial	Physical
Total =	Total =	Total =	Total =	Total =	Total =	Total =	Total =
Total ÷ 5 =	Total ÷ 5 =	Total ÷ 5 =	Total ÷ 5 =	Total ÷ 5 =	Total ÷ 5 =	Total ÷ 5 =	Total ÷ 5 =

(Add all 8 totals and divide the sum by 8 to get your IWQ) Total= _____ ÷ 8 = _____

At the end of this workbook I will invite you to measure your IWQ again and assess the difference in your scores. I encourage you to do an audit of your wellness twice a year or more often to address the areas you need to improve in your life and increase your IWQ. Remember, we are social beings, and relationships define our life's journey.

Questions

What will your relationships tell about how well you journey through this life?

_____

_____

Were your scores surprising or disappointing in any way?

_____

Would you like to set a goal to improve the above areas of your life?

_____

_____

How satisfied are you with the relationships in your life?

_____

_____

Here is a recap of the areas we will continue to focus on:

___ Spiritual/core values/self-esteem
___ Social/family relationship(s)
___ Emotional/stress
___ Occupational/career satisfaction
___ Intellectual/knowledge & skills
___ Environment/diversity and social impact
___ Financial/money/debt/planning
___ Physical/health
___ Interpersonal/collaboration

Questions

What are the obstacles or barriers to improving your IWQ score?

_____

_____

What is one thing you can do in the next 24 hours that will get you closer to your ideal score?

_____

_____

How might this change how others respond to you?

_____

_____

In addition to your Personal Wellness audit, what else can you do to help shed light on areas of your life that may need improvement?

_____

_____

If you are not happy with your score, I would like to ask that you acknowledge where you are now, appreciate your reality and celebrate where you intend to go.

Take some time to begin formulating a goal for your IWQ improvement.

My IWQ Improvement Goals:

_____

_____

_____

Personal Wellness Audit

Personal Wellness Audit (PWA) refers to the personal assessment you did in each dimension of your life. This exercise is designed to help you grasp the significance your daily choices and personal actions have on each area of your life and on the relationships in your life or work.

We are always creating, through our actions or inaction. We create a void by our lack of action. The universe requires all of us to create something as payment for our time here. When we cease to create, we are in essence denying who we are and what we are meant to do. By not doing, we become inert.

Please complete the exercises below to assess whether or not you are utilizing your capacity to create the things you desire in your life.

Questions

How does it feel to consider yourself as having the capacity to create or contribute?

_____

_____

Will this concept change the way you make choices, act or not act?

_____

A Personal Wellness Audit helps us to acknowledge our current reality and plan for the next step, where we want to go. Before we start setting goals for the future, it is important for us to take time to celebrate our present reality, because it represents what we have created in the past.

When we acknowledge and make peace with our present reality, we will gain the assurance required to assess our creativity and future possibilities without limits.

Reflect on your IWQ

What did you learn from doing your Personal Wellness audit?

_____

_____

Have you been able to grasp the significance of letting any one area of your life fall into disrepair?

_____

_____

Would it benefit you to improve your wellness in any of the dimensions or areas immediately? If so, which dimension or area and why?

_____

_____

What concerns or stressful thoughts arise when you think of doing a Personal Wellness audit twice a year?

_____

_____

How often would you prefer to do your Personal Wellness Audit and why?

_____

_____

Changing Your IWQ

Change in your IWQ will only occur if you become dissatisfied with the results of your current score and decide to change your reality. This means you will acknowledge the areas that are functioning well, recognize the areas that need further development, and become motivated and enthused to grow and develop these lesser-functioning areas to optimize the success of your relationships and improve your IWQ.

According to the IWS model concept, those who feel great will make others feel great, thereby impacting their wellness and stimulating a network of interpersonal wellness, which in turn results in a high IWQ and relationship success.

Questions

Are there times when you desire to make others feel great? When is this most likely?

_____

_____

What might you do to experience this feeling more often?

_____

_____

Are you happy with the areas of your life that are working well? Have you celebrated your success in those areas? How did you celebrate?

_____

_____

Personal Investment

Improving your IWQ or any other area of your life is a personal investment. Your life will only be richer from your efforts to invest in yourself. Investments should take patience and dedication and small or large deposits on a consistent basis. Ideally, we should commit to investing 15 to 30 minutes a day toward developing our personal wellness in each of the

eight life dimensions in order to maintain a great IWQ. Those who invest 30 to 60 minutes will see their level of success multiply at an exceptional rate, and an increase in their IWQ.

Questions

How much time can you invest in the next day/week to reflect on the areas of your life you want to recreate?

What changes in your life would result in more time and commitment to developing your IWQ?

_____

_____

_____

Your Personal Wellness Commitment

Plan to spend time each day developing your wellness in at least one area. Begin with five minutes and increase it by adding 5 minutes as you get more excited about the progress you see. I believe that it won't be long before you begin to dedicate 5 minutes or more to each area of your life, as you open yourself up to seeing the limitless possibilities ahead.

Questions

What is your personal time commitment for daily personal improvement?

_____

If you were to start with 5 minutes a day for Personal Wellness improvement, what do you think your result would be in 30 days?

_____

_____

_____

Gratifirmations

This is not a typo! It is a new word I created to refer to the act of practicing grateful affirmations for the things you believe yourself ready to receive. Later in this workbook, I discuss affirmations, but first, I want you to focus on the practice of gratifirmations as a way to help you begin acting as if that which you prayed or asked for is on its way. Remember, faith and works go together.

This practice lets you experience sensations of joy, fulfillment and gratitude, while you wait or take the necessary actions to create your new life reality.

I started practicing gratifirmations about four years ago, as a way to manifest the things I want in my life, and have had wonderful results. I also noticed that whenever I ceased this practice, the things I don't want, begin to come into my life. So here is how it works. You imagine yourself having obtained what you desire, then summon all the anticipated emotions and gratitude, plus more, and give all the thanks and gratitude you can muster.

Here is Jack's Gratifirmations

When Jack reflected on his IWQ of 4.75, as outlined in the introduction chapter, he was not thrilled with his capacity to contribute to his life relationships, so he wrote the following gratifirmations.

I am grateful that I have an IWQ of 7.4. I am grateful that this level of wellness has brought into my life a renewed relationship with my ex-wife, and meaningful conversations with my teenage sons. I am also grateful that this new level of wellness has aided in my developing a more enhanced working relationship with my supervisor. We are no longer in conflict and we spend time collaborating our energies to improve the company's service record. There is no longer distrust and negative competition between us.

I am grateful that I have now lost 15lbs, feel great and have a lot of energy and pizzazz. This has allowed me to take walks every evening-a refreshing part of my day. I am grateful that I now have an abundance of energy and I feel secure in both my personal and professional relationships. I am grateful that I have the confidence that I will be able to deal with whatever life may bring my way.

Now it's your turn. Find a quiet spot to reflect on your IWQ score from earlier. Think of the areas you want to make changes to and the ones that are doing well. Write out a gratifirmations like Jack's for each area or dimension where you want to have improved wellness. This simple exercise is very powerful and fulfilling. It also allows you to prevent or even stop worries and anxieties, as well as help you to manage fears about how you are

going to attain your new level of wellness. This practice will yield a higher level of consciousness to aid you in developing the vibrant pictures and pleasant sensations for holding your belief or faith. This will enthuse, motivate and sustain you on the path to your goals.

In the space below, take some time to write your own IWQ gratifirmations. Write out gratifirmations each day for six weeks as part of your daily prayer and devotion (especially in the early mornings) and it will help you to tap into the wonderful source of blessings that are ours for the asking.

Your IWQ Gratifirmations

_____

_____

_____

_____

_____

_____

_____

_____

_____

_____

_____

Notes

_____

_____

_____

He who is unable to live in society, or who has no need because he is sufficient for himself, must be either a beast or a god.

-Aristotle

A Time to Go Inside Self

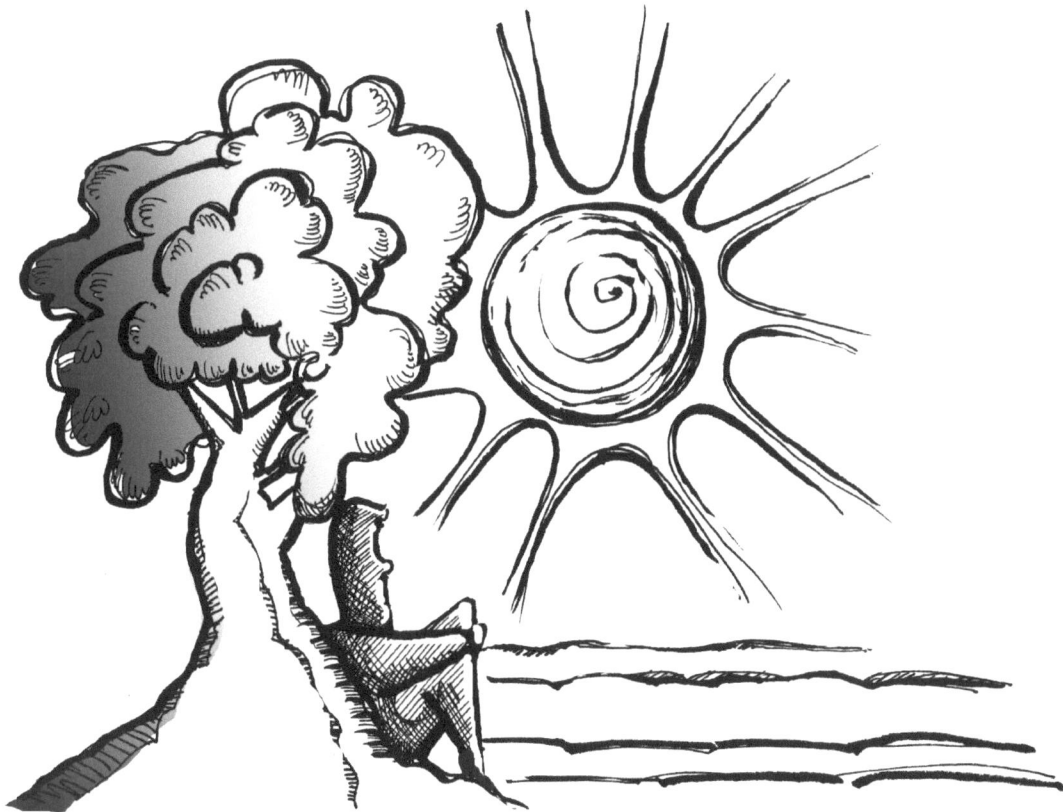

Spiritual

Every time you don't follow your inner guidance, you feel a loss of energy, loss of power, a sense of spiritual deadness.

-Shakti Gawain

Spiritual Dimension

Have you explored the potential benefits of having inner peace? Do you wonder how well you are experiencing and appreciating life and the natural forces that exist in our universe? Knowledge of how well you are doing in this dimension will help you advance. It is "a time to go inside" and reflect on the things that make up the core of who you are and what you want to give to the world.

Ask yourself, am I doing a well as I know I can in this area? If not how is this affecting my relationship with myself, my loved ones or co-workers?

In this chapter, I would like you to focus on the spiritual dimension of your life. Consider those things that make up the core of who you are. Reflect on the components that make up your spiritual wellness such as core values, trust, faith, prayer, beliefs, inspiration, integrity, culture, balance and self-esteem.

You are welcome to add or replace areas not listed above that you feel are of importance for your spiritual growth and wellness. Take this time to develop in this dimension as it will contribute to the furtherance of your IWQ. You have the capacity to make whatever change you believe needs to be made, if you exercise faith.

Let's look at how Jane changed her IWQ and as a result, changed her life. Jane was not happy with her life or relationships. She felt she needed to do something to improve her spiritual wellness and she selected to work on her core values. While doing this, she also worked on accountability from the intellectual dimension, social responsibility under the environmental dimension, rest under the physical dimension, and joy under the emotional dimension. She found that these things complemented each other and she reported noticing a rise in her IWQ. She now feels able to take on changes and growth in other areas. Jane plans to assess her IWQ every six months and work on at least five things, wherever necessary.

Assessing your Spiritual Wellness

To assess your spiritual wellness, please transfer the scores from your IWQ assessment. You may want to choose different areas from the previous ones you assessed.

What areas did you assess?

_____

_____

What have you noticed about your scores?

_____

_____

What is your spiritual wellness score? _____

How long have you been scoring this number? _____

Has your life situation changed recently in any of the categories?

_____

_____

Looking ahead, what score would you like to have for spiritual wellness? _____

What makes this your ideal spiritual wellness score? _____

_____

_____

How would you like to improve your wellness in this dimension?

_____

_____

How do you rate your likelihood of success in these areas?

_____

_____

What is one thing you might need to do to get you off to a good start?

_____

_____

Going Forward

Your personal audit in the spiritual dimension requires you to look inside yourself to discover who you really are and what beliefs motivate your actions. This will require you to do some personal inventory of what you believe about yourself, what inspires you, and in what or whom you have faith. This process will assist you in assessing your true values and the strength of your personal integrity.

Spirituality in this sense is much more than religious faith or denominational membership. Spirituality forms the essence of who we are and what motivates us. It is at the core of spirituality that we encounter our self-esteem. This determines what we believe about ourselves without external influence. It affects our personality, faith, choices, beliefs, value system, ability to find balance and our personal integrity.

Questions

As you think about this broad meaning of spiritual wellness, what comes to mind?

_____

_____

What are some things you have done in the past that have sustained your spiritual wellness?

_____

_____

What do you need to do more of to maintain spiritual wellness?

_____

_____

Is there a person, group, belief or attitude that is sabotaging your spiritual wellness?

_____

_____

Beliefs

Beliefs lie at the core of who we are. It is difficult for us to change our beliefs about ourselves or the things we hold dear without a change in perspective. We are at times bogged down by beliefs we were not aware we had, some are even damaging to our personal growth and development, causing fear in us that is unsubstantiated. It is important to examine our beliefs from time to time to see whether they are working for us or against us. See how Jane's belief directed her life.

Jane believed she was ugly, and so she wore unattractive clothing, did nothing with her hair and wore far too much makeup. She spoke passively, seldom made eye contact, did not interact well with others and took no initiative at work. As a result, she had few friends, no job promotions and minimal salary increases in her ten year career. Co-workers tended to avoid her and did not seek her opinion or give her a second glance. Jane was unaware of the negative impact her belief and choices were having on her life. She often said that people didn't like "ugly people" and she felt and sounded like a victim of her circumstances.

Jane was referred to coaching by her supervisor because she swore at a co-worker whom she claimed was disrespecting her. In coaching, she came to realize that her beliefs did guide her choices, which were responsible for the consequences she was facing. With this new insight, she experienced a shift in her perspective regarding beliefs, self-image and her choices of interpersonal interactions, dress and make-up. This was the beginning of her awareness and consequent behaviour change.

When asked how she would act if she thought of herself as beautiful, Jane came alive with ideas and possibilities. In this new reality, she found ways to change her actions and to positively change the effect she was having on others and within herself.

Jane now experiences a very different work reality. She interacts well with co-workers, wears the appropriate clothing and make-up and she is popular and well respected for her contributions at work. She has had a promotion and is on her way to becoming supervisor of her area.

Questions

What thoughts and beliefs might be controlling your actions and experiences?

_____

_____

What beliefs do you hold about your culture, values, integrity, faith or personal style?

_____

_____

Which core belief keeps you centred or grounded?

_____

_____

If you had to change one specific belief, which would it be, and why?

_____

_____

How might changing this belief improve other areas of your life?

_____

_____

What results do you anticipate?

_____

_____

What challenges would you face?

_____

_____

What broad ideas motivate you to change or not change that belief?

_____

_____

Have you found any evidence to support this belief?

_____

_____

How do these beliefs influence your actions?

_____

_____

How long have you acted on these beliefs?

_____

_____

How different would you be without these beliefs?

_____

_____

What new belief could you hold as a replacement to the ones you have identified?

_____

_____

What new realities would you like to picture for yourself?

_____

_____

Have you prayed or meditated on this desired change?

_____

_____

Building Trust

Trust is built over time, and is earned through self-confidence and consistent, reliable actions that show others we believe in ourselves and in our ability to be held accountable when necessary. Our assurance, coupled with consistent follow-through, helps others to believe in us, and over time they develop a sense of safety based on the reliability of our actions, which leads to trust.

Note that trust requires us to take some action, either to believe that one is able to earn trust or to acknowledge someone's effort to earn it. There is also the requirement for the person who wants to earn trust to take consistent action and to believe themselves capable of reliable and consistent actions. Here is how Jack and his wife are working on building trust.

Jack has been telling lies to his wife Jane about his spending habits for the last five years. When she finally found out about the state of their financial affairs, she told him she was no longer able to trust him. Jack is feeling devastated by his failure, but more so by the lack of trust in his intimate relationship. Jack knows that he has to work to earn Jane's trust again, so he is willing to tell the truth on a consistent basis regardless of the consequences.

Jane knows that in order to repair their relationship she needs to grow to trust Jack again. She is now acknowledging Jack's efforts to tell the truth and has made an effort to begin hoping that he will be truthful.

Questions

Are you ready to develop or rebuild trust in a relationship?

_____

_____

What is one action you can confidently take that would demonstrate responsibility?

_____

_____

What actions might you need to take to increase your consistency and reliability?

_____

_____

What action(s) can you take in the next week to rebuild trust in your relationship?

_____

_____

Faith

Trust comes before faith. It is not possible to have faith in something or someone we can't trust. One can have practical faith or religious faith, which is evidence of things hoped for but not seen. In Christian faith for example, Christians believe that the evidence of Christ having lived on earth gives them confidence to hope for His return and their ascension to Heaven.

We can also put our trust in a person and have faith that they will or will not do something. We can put faith in a partner's loyalty. It is often wise to have the person demonstrate an ability to be responsible and accountable before we put our trust or faith in them.

Questions

In whom do you put your faith?

_____

_____

Do you have a religious faith and does it give you peace?

_____

_____

What is your source of peace?

_____

_____

Do you have certain requirements as a basis for putting faith in someone or something?

_____

_____

Prayer or Meditation

When we really want something, we pray, meditate or dream that it will come true. Prayer and meditation have been proven to be great ways to go inside the self to assess what we really are grateful for. It is a time to quiet the mind and focus on the part of us that is unseen, untouched and often forgotten in the constant bustle of life.

Everyone can benefit from prayer or meditation, irrespective of what higher power we meditate upon or extend gratitude and adoration to.

Questions

Do you spend time in prayer of gratitude or meditation?

_____

_____

Do you meditate on your gifts, both what you have now and the things you hope to have in the future?

_____

_____

Do you spend time contemplating the skills and competencies you would like to develop?

_____

_____

What else can you pray for or meditate on to help you develop your spiritual wellness?

_____

_____

Personal Style

It is possible that you may have done a psychological analysis, personality tests or style assessment in the past. This would have introduced your dominant style, such as is commonly done with tools such as DISC or Myers Briggs.

This kind of typology categorizes you into a main group with certain tendencies and traits and helps you understand why or what to expect from those in a particular category. It also helps us better understand some unexplained tendencies or traits more fully. We are told that we develop style preferences through genetics and life shaping experiences and by learning.

Though we are unable to change our styles, we can learn new skills and techniques to manage our responses and impact on those in our interpersonal network.

IWQ is different from typologies assessments in that it helps you to identify your current areas of challenge regardless of your type. It focuses on one's current state, realizing that this is not a permanent state but one that can be improved or further neglected. The IWQ stems from a philosophy that every person can learn new skills and take actions to change their life realities and improve to contribute more meaningfully to their relationships.

Those who work in teams and groups or live in families may find this approach to be of great help in creating more opportunities for collaboration and Interpersonal Wellness.

Questions

Are you aware of your personal style or personality type?

_____

_____

Are you aware of how others experience this in your interactions?

_____

_____

According to Gilmore/Fraleigh's style profile assessment, we tend to have excesses in areas where we are strongest. Previously, these may have been identified as weaknesses. However, they believe that one can easily go into excess in an area of strength if awareness is not raised and proper self-management strategies are not executed. I also believe that it is important to continue learning and developing new skills in order to have a positive impact on others.

Remember that you are more than your style. Many factors will affect your style on a daily basis. Knowing and understanding your personal style will help you to develop proper self management strategies. In turn, this will enable you to experience your best self and greatly improve your IWQ.

Self-Management

Self-management or personal mastery is the art of understanding yourself and your strengths and excesses (the things you do too much of). It is learning how to reduce those negative impacts of your excesses. This is a responsibility we each have to ourselves and those in our life.

Self-management is a personal decision to assess, become self-aware and take responsibility to address our shortcomings. Self-management requires that we identify areas for growth and new learning that might help us see our situations and realities in a different context.

Many individuals learn self-management strategies through working with a coach. Others may develop this on their own or by working with another professional.

Self-management strategies can take the form of improved communication, being more attentive, learning to collaborate, being more responsible, breaking a bad habit, learning to say no, becoming aware of a bad attitude and changing the action, learning to negotiate or paying more attention to others.

Questions

If you completed a personal style assessment before, did you identify self- management strategies that could improve your positive impact on others?

_____

_____

What self-management strategies will you use to manage your excesses?

_____

_____

_____

What supports will you need to help you maintain this personal commitment?

_____

_____

_____

What is one strategy you can apply immediately?

_____

_____

What is one area in which you will need to develop new skills for better self- management?

_____

_____

_____

Values

The *New Webster* dictionary describes values as: "those things of worth, merit or importance to each of us, the ideas and beliefs we hold as special." Caring for others, for example, is a value.

We all have things that are of importance to us. When we live in disharmony with our true values and core beliefs, we are likely to feel disconnected with ourselves and with those in our relationships. This is because we no longer have a true source from which to contribute and participate in life.

When we have values that we live by, we become more principled in our approach to life. We are better equipped to set goals and to reach them successfully.

Questions

What are your values and how do your choices align with them?

_____

_____

Do you value love, peace, hard work, enthusiasm, solitude, what else?

_____

_____

What are some other values you hold? List your top ten values below:

1. _____

2. _____

3. _____

4. _____

5. _____

6. _____

7. _____

8. _____

9. _____

10. _____

What is most revealing about your list of values?

_____

_____

_____

What do you think these values say about you and your life?

_____

_____

_____

Are your daily actions in line with your top 5 values?

_____

_____

_____

How often do you make choices that have caused you distress or regret because you have compromised one of your values?

_____

_____

We should be making choices daily to live in alignment with our values, if not we will end up with regrets and disappointments.

The next time you set a goal, be sure to assess how it relates to one or more of your top ten values.

Self-esteem

Our spirit is directly related to our self-esteem. This is the part of us responsible for inspiration, development of core values and that motivates our quality of life. It is where we develop a picture of our self and our self-worth unfettered by outside influence.

In his book, *The Six Pillars of Self Esteem,* Dr. Nathanial Branden indentifies these six areas essential for the development and fostering of self-esteem: They are:

- Living consciously
- Self-acceptance
- Self-responsibility
- Self-assertiveness
- Living purposefully
- Personal integrity

I would like to expand on these and share the interpersonal wellness coaching perspective on how to help you apply these concepts to your own life and to rebuild or improve your own self-esteem.

Practising Conscious Living

I believe conscious living is a necessary element of Interpersonal Wellness. It requires you to take time to be aware of the details in your life, like the flowers you pass on a walk, your spouse's smile, a neighbour's friendly nature, and challenges that you encounter each day. This would require you to ask and answer the following questions:

What should I be learning today about myself?

_____

_____

What is one thing I learned today that I can grow from?

_____

_____

What things in my life do I need to take time to appreciate or acknowledge?

_____

_____

How might living consciously change my reality?

_____

_____

Practising Self-acceptance

This is another aspect of personal wellness that does impact your Interpersonal Wellness. When we practise self-acceptance, we also practise Responsible Communication (RC). This means that we will be open and honest in our actions. We guard our minds against negative self-talk and thoughts that may cause us to harbour beliefs detrimental to our wellness.

Questions

What thoughts are you harbouring that may be a detriment to your well-being?

_____

_____

Are there people in your close personal network who accept you as you are?

_____

_____

What is one action you are currently taking that is denying your self-acceptance?

_____

_____

What is one thing you can do to help improve your practise of self-acceptance?

_____

_____

Practising Self-responsibility

Self-responsibility reminds us that we are responsible for the choices we make as well as their consequences. Since we established that we create our own reality, it is imperative that we no longer see ourselves as victims or unlucky, but rather as reaping unsuspecting consequences. This then makes it necessary for us to take action to change our realities.

Questions:

Is there something in your life that you don't think you should be responsible for?

_____

_____

Is there an area in your life where you take full responsibility?

_____

_____

What is one action you can take to show more responsibility?

_____

_____

What can you do to change the results you are having in a particular area of your life?

_____

_____

Practising Self-assertiveness

When we practise self-assertiveness, we share ourselves with others in a respectful and honest way. We refrain from idle chatter, gossip and negativity about ourselves and others. We show courage and take a stand for the things we believe in an appropriate way. We also trust that if we make a mistake we can own up to it and take corrective action. The practice of self-assertiveness will greatly impact our IWQ by building trust in ourselves and with others.

Questions:

Is there an area in your life where you need to respectfully take a stand?

_____

_____

Is there an area in your life where you need to be more positive and affirming?

_____

_____

Is there an area in your life where you need to own up to a mistake and begin corrective actions?

_____

_____

Practising Purposeful Living

Living a purposeful life is akin to living successfully. Those who live with purpose often have high rates of success in their lives and relationships. It is important to ensure that you are living in a meaningful and purposeful way in all dimensions of your life as reflected in the IWS model. An individual will be okay in the short term with deficits in one or more dimensions, but over time it is important not to over-compensate in any one dimension in hopes that it will balance out the others.

Each dimension of your life deserves purposeful attention and development to keep functioning optimally.

Questions

Is there an area of your life where you think you need to develop more meaning and purpose?

_____

_____

What would that look like for you and how would this change your life?

_____

_____

What helps you to be successful in maintaining meaning and purpose in your life?

_____

_____

Practising Personal Integrity

To practise personal integrity is to live in congruence with the values we hold true. This does not mean you should live by values someone else holds or may try to impose on you. Each of us has the right to decide what is important to us and what standards we will honour. Our integrity comes into question when our actions are incongruent with our commitments. In order to maintain a healthy IWQ, it is important for us to be clear about our values. This makes it possible for others to hold us accountable when our actions don't reflect our stated values.

Questions

What is one thing that helps you to maintain personal integrity in your life?

_____

_____

Do you wrestle with issues around personal responsibility and low self-esteem?

_____

_____

Which of the 6 pillars of self-esteem discussed above did you find most informative and insightful?

_____

_____

What would your life be like if you were to successfully work through these areas?

_____

_____

Visualization

Someone once said that everything begins with a thought. Visualization is a wonderful gift that allows us to step away from our current situation and envision what we want to accomplish in the future. This allows us to focus on the important steps we need to take to maintain a healthy IWQ. When we visualize, we create an image that keeps us enthused into action to create what we have visualized.

Visualization is different from dreaming. While we may dream about something for a long time and take no action towards reaching that dream, visualization is purposeful in that it is done to help us develop a road map or image of something we intend to create.

Questions

What new reality do you visualize for yourself?

_____

_____

Have you come up with a plan on how to create this new image?

_____

_____

What resources and support will you need to create the life you visualized?

_____

_____

All human actions have one or more of these seven causes: chance, nature, compulsion, habit, reason, passion, and desire.

-Aristotle

Chapter Insight

As you look back on the readings and exercises in this chapter, what insights have you gained? What aspects were of most importance to you?

_____

_____

_____

_____

Please use the chart below to note your insights, the date and your intended actions. Three months from this date, please revisit this chart and note the steps you have taken.

Insight/Date	Intended Action Step	Complete 0-100%
1		
2		
3		

Reflections

What is one thing you experienced from this spiritual dimension chapter that changed your focus or thinking?

_____

_____

How much responsibility do you believe you have over your feelings and experiences?

_____

_____

What belief or judgment will you now put away?

_____

_____

What new structures have you been able to put in place to support future growth in the spiritual dimension of your life?

_____

_____

Notes

_____

_____

_____

_____

So divinely is the world organized that every one of us, in our place and time, is in balance with everything else.

-Johann Wolfgang von Goethe

A Time to Build Community

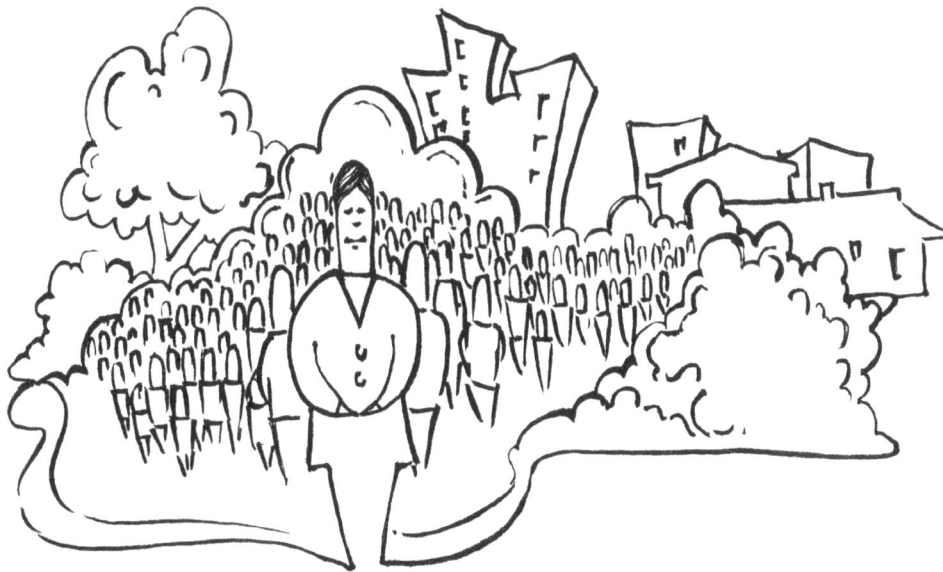

Social

Call it a clan, call it a network, call it a tribe, call it a family. Whatever you call it, whoever you are, you need one.

-Jane Howard

Social Dimension

Have you explored the potential benefits of having a great social network? Do you wonder how well others are experiencing you? I consider this "a time to build community". This means that it is never too late to change how others will experience you in the future.

Ask yourself, am I doing a well as I know I can in this area? If not, how is this affecting my relationship with my loved ones or co-workers?

The interpersonal relationships that comprise our social network can include work teams and colleagues, family, church or club members, or our neighbours. Our relationships with individuals in these groups will be impacted by our level of personal wellness in each dimension and will directly determine our IWQ. Our ability to form healthy social relationships and communicate responsibly is a key to our personal and professional success, and this determines the life we are able to create and realize.

Organizations want to hire individuals who have good interpersonal skills. The exercises in this section, like in the rest of this workbook will help you develop your skills into interpersonal competencies, allow you to improve your IWQ and realize optimal success in your career.

Assessing your Social Wellness

To assess your social wellness, please transfer the scores from your IWQ assessment. You may want to assess different areas from the ones you assessed previously.

What areas did you assess?

_____

_____

What have you noticed about your scores?

_____

_____

What is your social wellness score? _____

How long have you been scoring this number? _____

Has your life situation changed recently in any of these areas? If so which one, and how?

_____

_____

Looking ahead, what score would you like to have for social wellness? _____

What makes this your ideal social wellness score? _____

_____

_____

How would you like to improve your social dimension?

_____

_____

How do you rate your likelihood of improving your wellness in these areas?

_____

_____

What is one thing you might need to do to get you off to a good start?

_____

_____

Blind Spots

We all have flaws in our own characters. Some of us are aware of these, while others have no idea that they exist. When we don't know they exist, we refer to them as blind spots. Most times, these will be identified by working with a coach or by gaining feedback from those with whom we interact closely.

Obtaining feedback is a rewarding, awareness-raising exercise that helps us to grow. It also helps us to become aware of things we had not even considered and it increases our interpersonal intelligence, so we can make informed decisions about how to improve our ability to contribute to the wellness of our relationships – our IWQ.

To do this, you are required to ask three people whom you trust, either at home, work, school or your church, to give you truthful feedback when filling out the Personal Feedback Questionnaire in appendix A. You can also access this on our website by going to www.interpersonalwellness.com/bookresources and click on the link the Personal Feedback Questionnaire.

Please remind those you've chosen that this exercise is for awareness-raising and personal development work, and is imperative that they not spare your feelings but be honest about what they have observed about you.

Please provide a photocopy of the questionnaire from appendix A to the individuals you have selected for their feedback. Good Luck!

Obstacles to Change

Competition and the struggle to come out ahead have helped to eradicate feelings of interdependence in the workplace. Many employees complain of back-biting, gossiping, ambiguity and lack of trust as their greatest sources of stress at work. As a result, they wear masks or social identities they find necessary for self- preservation.

This masking of self has led to larger problems, such as disconnection with self and others, resulting in a lack of personal responsibility and accountability. The ensuing rise in interpersonal conflicts and recurring disputes in the workplace have been identified as further evidence of this.

Questions

Do you feel vulnerable or unsafe at work? If so, has this been a long-term issue or is it recent?

_____

_____

Is there a mask, or self, you use for work that helps you to feel safe?

_____

_____

Those who have developed negative social identities tend to find they are unable to move out of that role. The inflexibility of those in our social groups, such as family, colleagues, community or workplace, can negatively influence our personal growth. These inflexible attitudes have the potential to keep one in a mould that may discourage growth and change.

Comments such as "Jane will never change" would make changing her behaviour challenging, without the support of a coach to encourage her to take new actions and develop structures to sustain her new skills.

Negative beliefs and self-talk may be generated from inflexible attitudes that cause one to make comments such as: "I can't do that; no one will expect me to act that way." Often individuals who have earned a negative reputation based on past actions and behaviours relay these self-defeating comments.

Questions

Do you think that you are worthy of a new positive belief about your behaviour? Why or why not?

_____

_____

Do you think it's time to find out who you really are? Yes or no? _____

What belief controls your thoughts and your actions?

_____

_____

What is the worst possible thing that could go wrong, if you were to adopt a new belief?

_____

_____

I encourage you to contemplate your answers to those questions. It is my hope that they will motivate you to become more self-directing, self-correcting and self-generating in your future actions. This may be your time to grab hold of what you are worth and accept nothing less!

Status

Each of us has earned a certain social status in our group, family or workplace within which we wield a certain level of influence. Often we abuse, dismiss or are ignorant of our social influence. When we are fully conscious of our status and the responsibilities that it brings, we are much more likely to practise Responsible Communication.

In so doing, we will make intelligent decisions about what we say yes or no to, as well as what we discuss and the social vibrations we generate. We will also be certain that we speak in a clear, direct manner that reflects self-awareness and confidence.

Networking

Everyone has a network. This may not be huge or extensive but if you look around you will find that you have a group of people you belong to, are a part of or engage with. This comprises your network. Too often we go through life not realizing just how extensive our network may be and just who we may be able to actually network with. I think it is a real shame when we go through life dejected and alone rather than looking for ways to expand our network and share ourselves with others. Life is about relationships and humans are in the relationship business. Without people, it is impossible for this world to continue. Why not take some time to look around you and assess your current network and see how you can trade, barter services or negotiate for resources within your network.

Questions

Are you aware of your social status in your work or family group?

_____

_____

Do you think your status lends you a measure of influence at home or at work?

_____

_____

Who might be influenced by you?

_____

_____

_____

Responsible Communication

Responsible Communication (RC) requires that you practise collaborative dialogue. To do this, one needs to demonstrate respect, attention, voicing, listening and silence as a way to communicate a desire to work in harmony. RC requires that you use tone, cadence and body language to show caring, courtesy and openness as well as a willingness to act responsibly in your choice of words and actions. Those who practise RC should also show a high sense of accountability for the consequences of their communication. RC requires good use of words and mannerisms and a desire to make a positive impact.

It is also demonstrated in one's willingness to clear up misunderstandings and apologize for any discomfort that was caused in the exchange.

Responsible Communication will exemplify the following elements:

- Being clear, direct, and purposeful about our communication

- Being accountable for the impact and consequences of what we communicate

- Ensuring that attitude, tone, cadence and words reflect a message for which we are willing to be held accountable

Collaborative Dialogue

In his book, *Teaching An Anthill to Fetch*, Stephen Joyce describes collaborative dialogue as four step process. I think it is really a five step process that comes together beautifully when people are able to think and work together. I will share them here as:

- Reciprocity
- Acknowledgement
- Inclusiveness
- Transparency
- Consultation

Reciprocity is the act of giving in kind. I have never been asked to intervene in a conflict situation where there is a perceived sense of reciprocity. When reciprocity is not practiced people get upset and there is an outcry for justice.

Acknowledgement is a very under-utilized interpersonal success strategy. If only we acknowledged and complemented each other's strengths and gifts rather than point out our weak spots, we would find that the world would be a much better place to live and people would be much happier.

Inclusiveness is the act of making others feel welcome and a part of our group, process or conversation. It could be a smile, eye contact or an inviting word. People usually fight to be included. No one likes to be excluded.

Transparency requires openness, clarity and accessibility. No one wants to be in a situation where there is a lack of clarity and confusion about what is happening. People get upset when they can't gain information.

Consultation is the process of gaining input from others. Too many change processes and project failure occur because of a lack of consultation. Consultation gains buy in and help to obtain participation. To launch a new venture without participation is risky.

These are important elements of responsible communication that work to create collaborative exchanges. If you practice these steps you will notice that others will want to collaborate with you.

Questions

How would you describe your level of Responsible Communication?

_____

_____

Are there areas where you would like to strengthen your communication?

_____

_____

Do you regularly take responsibility for what you communicate?

_____

_____

Do you try to be clear and respectful in your communication?

_____

_____

Boundaries

One of the most important aspects of the social dimension is the ability to set and maintain social boundaries. Boundaries define relationships and set parameters within which one acts and relates in any social interaction. They help to remove ambiguity by providing a framework for the relationship. Every healthy family, workplace or social group needs boundaries that define the relationship and structure the roles of those within it. The establishment of boundaries helps to reduce ambiguity and interpersonal conflicts. It also helps to clear up misunderstandings, intractable conflicts and unnecessary competition.

Boundaries provide a common understanding of what is appropriate in the relationship. They inform us of what is expected of us, and our responsibility to act within those parameters or be held accountable. It is also easier to resolve minor disputes and misunderstandings when there are known boundaries. It is easier to call someone's action into question and encourage one to be accountable if there is a common understanding of the expectations.

Questions

Do you have clearly established boundaries in your relationships, how are they maintained?

_____

_____

Is there a relationship where you need to reconsider your role, if so why?

_____

_____

What is one thing you can do to change your relationship today?

_____

_____

_____

_____

Are the boundaries in your relationship being respected?

_____

_____

Chapter Insight

As you look back on the readings and exercises in this chapter, what insights have you gained? What aspects were of most importance to you?

_____

_____

_____

_____

Please use the chart below to note your insights, the date and your intended actions. Three months from this date, please revisit this chart to note your level of completion.

Insight/Date	Intended Action/Step	Complete 0-100%
1		

2		
3		

Reflections

What is one thing you experienced in the social dimension that changed your focus or thinking?

_____

_____

How might you do things differently to change or enhance your social wellness?

_____

_____

What is one personal growth area you have identified and how will it help improve your IWQ?

_____

_____

What new structures have you been able to put in place to support your personal growth?

_____

_____

Notes:

_____

_____

_____

_____

To enjoy the things we ought and to hate the things we ought has the greatest bearing on excellence of character."

-Aristotle

A Time to Manage Self

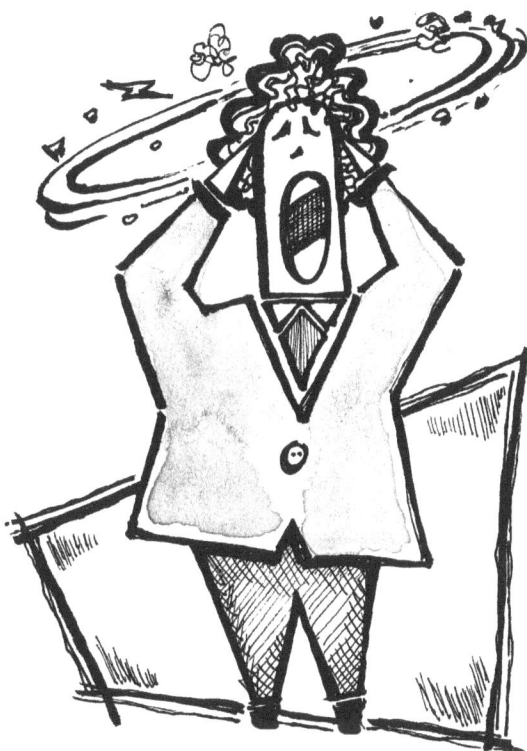

Emotional

Happiness cannot be traveled to, owned, earned, worn or consumed. Happiness is the spiritual experience of living every minute with love, grace and gratitude.
-Denis Waitley

Emotional Dimension

Have you explored the potential benefits of having great emotional balance? Do you wonder how much simpler your life could be if you had or practiced better emotional wellness? How are others experiencing your emotional turmoil, upset and anger? Does it make interacting with you difficult or pleasant? I consider this "a time to manage self". We can all do more to improve our emotional intelligence.

Ask yourself, am I doing a well as I know I can in this area? If not, how is this affecting my relationship with my loved ones or co-workers?

Emotional Intelligence (EQ) can be described as one's ability to understand and manage emotions. It is also the ability to correctly identify, assess and positively impact the emotions of those in your interpersonal network, thereby demonstrating your IWQ. Management of emotions is a social responsibility; we need to be more aware and assume more responsibility for the wellness of our relationships.

As we discussed earlier, we communicate and contribute in our relationships through social vibrations, as well as through our actions and words. This chapter will help you explore and identify your emotional management skills and provide a guide to help you develop your emotional wellness to positively impact your IWQ.

To manage self is to put in place a strategy to develop your emotional wellness as well as your IWQ. You can do this on your own or by working with a coach or other professional to develop your interpersonal skills and IWQ.

The following personal audit will help you to identify your score in the emotional dimension, where you can assess areas such as self-awareness, fear, anxiety, anger, joy, disappointment, resentment, doubt, regret, and the management of self.

Assessing your Emotional Wellness

To assess your emotional wellness, please transfer the scores from your IWQ assessment. You may want to assess different areas from those you have assessed earlier.

Do you consider yourself to have a high emotional wellness? If yes, how high is it? If low, do you want to improve it?

_____

_____

Do you believe that you have a social responsibility to improve your emotional wellness?

_____

_____

What areas of your emotional dimension did you assess?

_____

_____

What have you noticed about your scores?

_____

_____

What is your emotional wellness score? _____

How long have you been scoring this number? _____

Has your life situation changed recently in any of these areas, if so which one, and how?

_____

_____

Looking ahead, what score would you like to have for emotional wellness? _____

What makes this your ideal emotional wellness score?

_____

_____

_____

How would you like to improve your emotional dimension?

_____

_____

How do you rate your likelihood of improving your emotional wellness?

_____

_____

What is one thing you might need to do to get you off to a good start?

_____

_____

See how Harriet Demonstrated Emotional Wellness

Harriet is responsible for collecting the mail at her workplace. On Mondays and Wednesdays the marketing department tends to have a high volume of mail, which makes it too heavy for Harriet to transport unaided. Her supervisor arranged to have Jim from the marketing department assist Harriet in transporting the mail on those days, but Jim seems unwilling to assist and often does so grudgingly. He usually makes snide remarks implying that Harriet is being a baby. Last Monday when he brought the mail down to the mailroom, he bumped his leg on a stool and yelled at Harriet, who was busy working at the other end of the room. She noted Jim's words and smiled at him, wishing him a good day. Jane, who happened to witness the exchange, was very upset and asked Harriet why she was being so nice to Jim. Harriet replied that she was not being nice to Jim but rather nice to herself, since she didn't think it was worth getting caught up in Jim's misery.

Questions

Do you think that Jim is managing emotions well?

_____

_____

Do you think that Harriet should have been angry with Jim for his rude behaviour?

_____

_____

What advice do you have for Jim?

_____

_____

Is Jim's language helping him to have a good work experience?

_____

_____

Do you think Jim is contributing positively to the wellness of this working relationship?

_____

_____

Someone once said that there are only two true emotions, fear and love. If we are to believe this, we would assume that emotions such as joy, anger, doubt, resentment, anxiety and the like, fall under one of these two categories.

Questions

Do you readily acknowledge and examine feelings of fear?

_____

_____

How do you express your feelings of fear?

_____

_____

If you were to acknowledge when you felt fear, might this change your relationships?

_____

_____

Is there a relationship in which you need to practice more consideration?

_____

_____

In the following exercise, I would like you to keep track of the emotions in your life and how you manage them versus how much they help you increase your level of interpersonal wellness at home or work.

Over the next 30 days, use the following worksheet to log how you are improving your emotional management. You may substitute the areas with choices more relevant to you.

Please indicate by how much your IWQ increased (+) based on your assessment on day 1 of keeping the log. You may keep track of emotions such as anger, fear, joy, disappointment, anxiety, doubt or any others relevant to you.

IWS Emotional Management Success Plan

	Self-Awareness	Self-Management	IWQ +
Day	A	B	C
1			
2			
3			
4			
5			
6			
7			
8			

9			
10			
11			
12			
13			
14			
15			
16			
17			
18			
19			
20			
21			
22			
23			
24			
25			
26			
27			
28			
29			
30			

Exploring Anger

Anger is a primary emotion that we are all capable of expressing in some form; however, the way you choose to express it can result in a lot of hurt and turmoil in your interpersonal relationships. Like other stressful emotions, anger is a sign that our needs are not being met or that we are hurt or fearful. To reduce angry outbursts, it is important to address each stressful situation rationally and logically and communicate your concerns in a non-threatening or non-judgmental way.

In this section, I will discuss some information about anger that may help you better manage your responses to anger.

Questions

Do you tend to show your feelings of anger in negative outbursts?

_____

_____

Do you believe that there is something you can do to better respond to anger?

_____

_____

Reasons for Anger

If you participated in a style profile assessment with your coach, you will now be able to identify the situations that drive you into excess. If you haven't yet completed an assessment then take some time to think about when you feel most angry and the reasons why you feel angry.

Let's take a look at four of the most common reasons people respond with anger:

1. **Feeling hurt:** when our feelings are hurt, it is easier to get angry at the person who has emotionally wounded us than it is to acknowledge the hurt.
2. **Feeling betrayed:** feelings of betrayal affect us deeply: often our instinctive response can be one of overwhelming anger at the person who has betrayed us.
3. **Feeling embarrassed:** responding with anger becomes a way of masking one's shame or embarrassment.
4. **Feeling threatened:** responding with anger to personal threat is one way to ensure that we preserve life and dignity.

Questions

What do you think are your top two reasons for feelings and expressions of anger at work?

_____

_____

Anger Management

Understanding what makes you angry is important in finding solutions to manage your anger. To interact successfully with others, it becomes necessary to learn ways of dealing with anger that are respectful of yourself and others.

Questions:

What are two things that make you angry at home?

_____

_____

Knowing this, what might you do differently the next time you feel yourself getting angry at a situation or person?

_____

_____

_____

_____

Would you like to change your anger response pattern?

_____

What is one thing that you can do in the next week that will help you feel successful in managing feelings of anger?

_____

_____

What kind of support or resources do you need to help you do this better?

_____

_____

Our Feelings and Anger

We all face fear, anxiety, resentment and regret from time to time. That is why it's important for us to learn skills that will help us to assess the negative thoughts and self talk that accompany these feelings. The following questions will help you investigate your thoughts and decide if they are real.

Questions

What are you most fearful of?

_____

_____

What would your life be like without these feelings of fear?

_____

_____

Do you feel injured, hurt or abused by someone or a situation?

_____

_____

What things or situations bring you peace and joy?

_____

_____

How are you limited by your feelings of fear or anxiety?

_____

_____

After reflecting on the discussion of anger in this chapter, please list below some strategies you will apply when dealing with your anger, and for responding to anger directed at you by someone else.

Anger Management Strategies

Strategies for dealing with my own anger	Strategies for dealing with another person's anger
•	•
•	•
•	•
•	•
•	•
•	•

Points to keep in mind:

- Others have a right to feel angry too. Anger is as valid an emotion as joy or grief.

- Anger is the body and mind's method of communicating extreme emotions or extreme discomfort.

- Aggressive actions by others may be a sign of fear or frustration.

- Avoid the bait! Know your own triggers and stay in an objective and neutral frame of mind (stay calm and focused on the problem). Think cooperation!

- Become a partner in the problem-solving process.

- Allow others to vent their anger before moving to a discussion. Your steps to discount or defend can only increase levels of distress.

- If the situation approaches violence, get help and/or remove yourself from the situation.

The Importance of Forgiveness

In the broad general sense, forgiveness is the decision to move past a hurt, injustice or painful experience that has caused you anger, resentment, disappointment, frustration, betrayal or the desire for revenge. This may include releasing ill will towards the person(s) who caused the hurt, even if it's you. It is the process of ceasing to feel resentment, indignation or anger for a perceived or real offense, or ceasing to demand punishment or restitution.

Forgiveness has no set pattern. Sometimes forgiveness comes after an apology has been extended and received. Other times it comes simply from a decision to let go of the pain, or from taking back your power and untying yourself from the perceptions and feelings that bind you to the perceived injustice. This can reduce the power these feelings have over you, so that you can live a happier, unrestrained life in the present. Forgiveness may even lead to feelings of understanding, empathy and compassion for the one who has hurt you.

It can also mean freeing yourself from the significance that was placed on the actions of the other person.

Questions

Are you curious to experience how forgiveness may bring you positive benefits?

_____

_____

What would your life be like if you did not have this feeling of resentment or fear?

_____

_____

_____

_____

Chapter Insight

As you look back on the readings and exercises in this chapter, what insights have you gained? What aspects were of most importance to you?

_____

_____

_____

Please use the chart below to note your insights, the date and your intended actions. Three months from this date, please revisit this chart to note your level of completion.

Insight/Date	Intended Action/Step	Complete 0-100%
1		
2		
3		

Reflections

What is one thing you experienced in the emotional dimension that changed your focus or thinking?

_____

_____

How might you do things differently to change or enhance your emotional wellness?

_____

_____

What is one personal growth area you have identified and how will it improve your IWQ?

_____

_____

What new structures have you been able to put into place to support your personal growth?

_____

_____

Are there areas in your life where you need to reconcile with the past and forgive yourself or someone in order to move forward?

_____

_____

Are there times when you have thought forgiveness would be good, but found yourself staying committed to the pain or hurt?

_____

_____

What role is fear of trusting again having on your ability to forgive?

_____

_____

What issues do you find most difficult to forgive?

_____

_____

What do you need to tell yourself to be able to reconcile the hurt?

_____

_____

What new habits will you need to develop and apply?

_____

_____

Identify one thing you can do to make this habit stick:

_____

Notes:

_____

_____

_____

_____

It is the nature of desire not to be satisfied, and most men live only for the gratification of it.

-Aristotle

A Time for Achievement

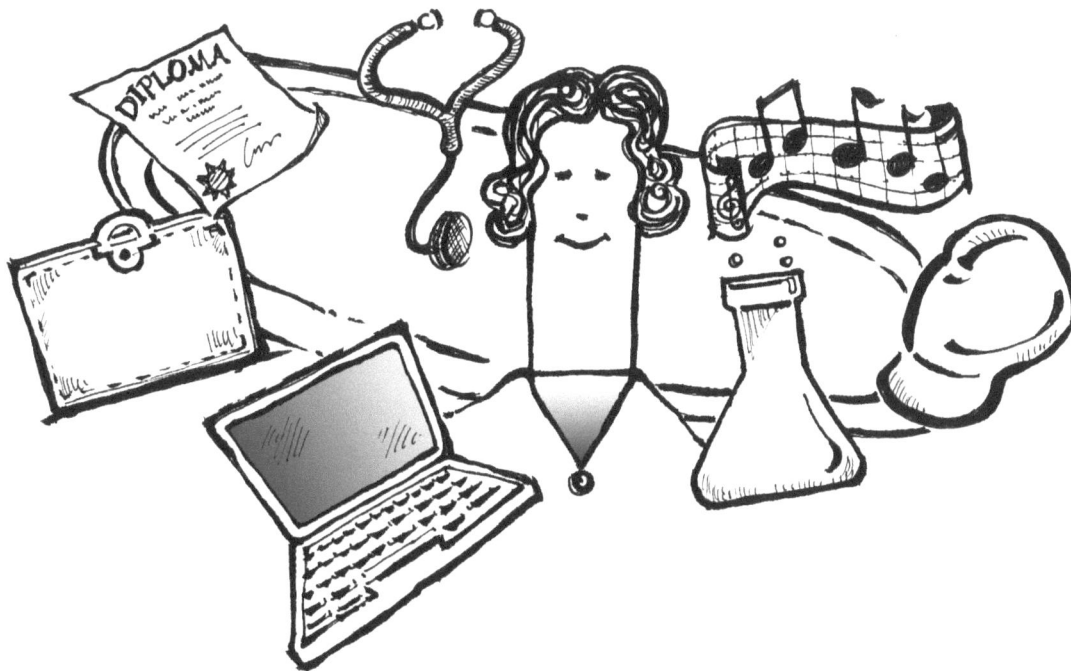

Occupational

It's not necessarily about what career you pick. It's about how you do what you do.

-Cory Doctorow

Occupational Dimension

Have you explored the potential benefits of having a great career and a healthy work environment? Do you wonder how well you are doing in career and working relationship? Imagine yourself in a beautiful job where you are making a positive impact on the world and contributing your skills to humanity. I consider this "a time to achieve". This is a great time to reflect on what you want to achieve professionally and what you need to do to reach your goal.

Ask yourself, am I doing a well as I know I can in this area? If not, how is this affecting my relationship with my loved ones or co-workers?

Our society has programmed us to believe that having an occupation in which we take pride and that holds certain esteem or status is a symbol of success.

Pride in one's job or occupation has been touted as the ultimate determinant of success. However, many individuals in the workplace declare unhappiness or dislike of their work situations mainly due to interpersonal conflicts or poor interactions. I often hear comments such as, "I like my job but not the people". Since most jobs require some interaction with people, it is essential that we learn to develop adequate interpersonal skills to manage good work situations but also to negotiate around the less than pleasant situations.

Self-employment is viewed as the ideal and many people express a desire to quit their jobs and work for themselves. It is sad to say that even in those cases they end up having difficulty negotiating with colleagues and business associates. It is not surprising that several poll results show that many people experience a very high level of stress relating to their occupation.

The World Health organization estimates that depression and coronary health disease will be the two highest causes of employee disability by 2020. In this chapter, I hope that you will take some time to reflect on what you bring to your job and how you can contribute positively towards making the working environment less stressful and safer for you and your colleagues.

Assessing your Occupational Wellness

To assess your occupational wellness, please transfer the scores from your IWQ assessment. You may want to assess different areas from the ones you previously assessed.

What areas did you assess?

_____

_____

What have you noticed about your scores?

_____

_____

What is your occupational wellness score? _____

How long have you been scoring this number? _____

Has your life situation changed recently in any of these areas, if so which one, and how?

_____

_____

Looking ahead, what score would you like to have for occupational wellness? _____

What makes this your ideal occupational wellness score? _____

_____

_____

How would you like to improve your occupational dimension?

_____

_____

How do you rate your likelihood of improving your wellness in these areas?

_____

What is one thing you might need to do to get you off to a good start?

_____

_____

Workplace Realities

Workplace conflicts are everywhere. Frequent misunderstandings, disagreements and disputes will help to deteriorate Interpersonal Wellness at work. As a matter of fact, when surveyed, many individuals identify work as the greatest source of their stress.

Many of us define ourselves by our occupation, and too often it becomes the umbrella under which we live our lives. Jane is a nurse and all her friends are nurses. She often makes nurse/patient jokes, and when asked if she wanted to join the local softball team, her first thought was "will there be other nurses on the team?"

Having things in common with co-workers are fine, but it's important to have a separation of work and personal life. When we limit our interactions to those within our professions, it's very easy for group think to set in, leaving us rigid, inflexible, closed and without fresh perspectives in our thinking and actions.

Questions

Do you define yourself by your occupation? _____

Do the majority of your friends have the same occupation as you do? _____

Occupation as Symbol of Financial Success

People often introduce themselves by their occupations-I'm a teacher, a lawyer, a life coach or a doctor-but what does that really say about who they are? Are they good people? Do they care about their clients or colleagues? Are they good parents or spouses? Do they care about the well-being of their patients, or are they in the profession because of the status and salary scale?

It is important to choose an occupation for which you have a passion or desire. This reduces burnout and work dissatisfaction.

We invest so much of our identity into our occupation that it is crucial to maintain a healthy IWQ in order to achieve balance at work. We also need to ensure that work does not become all-consuming; as we continually improve our IWQ contributions in personal and social relationships.

Since we spend the majority of our time at work, this may be why we identify ourselves by our occupations. Think of the last time you defined yourself by the experience you were having in a relationship or job. We should all work to be proud of our relationships at home and at work.

Questions

Do you invest the same amount of time in any other area of your life as you do in your occupation?

_____

_____

Do you take vacations and scheduled time off work?

_____

_____

How personally invested are you in your occupation?

_____

_____

What are some structures you use to separate your work life from your personal life?

_____

_____

Did you recently have a job transition or promotion?

_____

_____

What is currently the most difficult aspect of your job?

_____

_____

Work Stress

Most of the stress we have at work is related to beliefs we hold about our work, our colleagues, our roles or ourselves. These beliefs may stem from low job satisfaction, inadequate skills to manage new roles and responsibilities, or lack of support to develop skills into competencies to make our jobs less difficult.

Another main area of stress at work is poor problem-solving skills. Too often we blame and complain rather than focus on the issues at hand. Problem solving is practical and problem-focused. However, when problems arise and we engage in the blame game without thought, we miss out on great opportunities to engage others and harness the collective potential of a collaborative approach.

If we were to view our occupations as an opportunity to serve connect or become part of a community, that belief would motivate engaging thoughts and actions that would stimulate in us a higher sense of responsibility. We would then be more aware of our views, actions and interactions with others in our workplace, and create opportunities to do more, give more and strive for more, to become our very best self.

Questions

Are you in a high-stress occupation, if so, how stressful is it?

_____

_____

What stress management strategies do you use to cope with your work realities?

_____

_____

Does your occupation inspire you to grow or improve?

_____

_____

If you are unhappy with your current job or position, what are you doing about it?

_____

_____

What is one step you can take to help you get into the occupation you desire?

_____

_____

Is there a work relationship you need to improve?

_____

_____

Is there a resource at work that can aid you in managing your stress and career planning?

_____

_____

Jack's Career Growth

Jack was unhappy with his job as supervisor at the local shop yard. He believed that he had the capacity to work in a different profession. However, Jack had bills to pay and a family to support. When he learned that his local college provided distance learning courses he decided to try one course. He completed his course-work on his lunch breaks and did his readings on the bus to and from work. Five years later, Jack graduated with a diploma, which he later upgraded to degree and later an MBA.

Jack tells of his many long nights and the times when he considered giving up but, he kept his focus on completing one course at a time, and over time he had completed years of schooling. Looking back 10 years later, Jack recalls his progress and is proud of himself and the sacrifices he made even when it seemed hopeless all those years ago as struggled with his first course. Today, Jack is one of the managing directors of his company!

Questions

What is inspiring about Jack's path?

_____

_____

What would motivate you to go after your career dreams?

_____

_____

When was the last time you went after a dream? What structures and support helped you to succeed?

_____

_____

Healthy Work Environment

A healthy work environment is one in which there is collaboration, open dialogue, a commitment to wellness, a desire for healthy relationships, and a desire to reduce harm to each other. It is also an environment in which responsible communication is practiced and respect and dignity is expressed by employees and management alike.

Questions

How are you contributing to a healthy work environment?

_____

Is there an action or skill that may assist you in creating a healthier work environment?

_____

_____

Career Opportunities

Career opportunities are options to improve, expand or elevate your career within your current organization, your profession, industry or elsewhere. These are not always obvious and at times you will need to find or create these opportunities for yourself. This may mean, upgrading your skills, earning a professional designation, gaining experience, taking some courses or going back to school as a way to increase your credibility and marketability.

You may want to do something such as networking with those in your organization, an association you are a member of, through your roster or by volunteering. You will also need to do some research of the industry you want to work in to improve your chances of moving up the ladder. Ask yourself, what am I doing to advance my career opportunities?

Questions

What are your current career goals?

_____

_____

Is there a career opportunity you need to make happen for yourself?

_____

_____

Chapter Insight

As you look back on the readings and exercises in this chapter, what insights have you gained?

_____

_____

What aspects were of most importance to you?

_____

_____

Please use the chart below to note your insights, the date and your intended actions. Three months from this date, please revisit this chart to note your level of completion.

Insight/Date	Intended Action/Step	Complete 0-100%
1		
2		
3		

Reflections

What is one thing you experienced in the occupational dimension that changed your focus or thinking?

_____

_____

How might you do things differently to change or enhance your occupational wellness?

_____

_____

What is one personal growth area you have identified and how will it help improve your IWQ?

_____

What new structures have you been able to put in place to support your personal growth?

_____

_____

Notes

_____

_____

_____

_____

A likely impossibility is always preferable to an unconvincing possibility.

-Aristotle

A Time for Growth

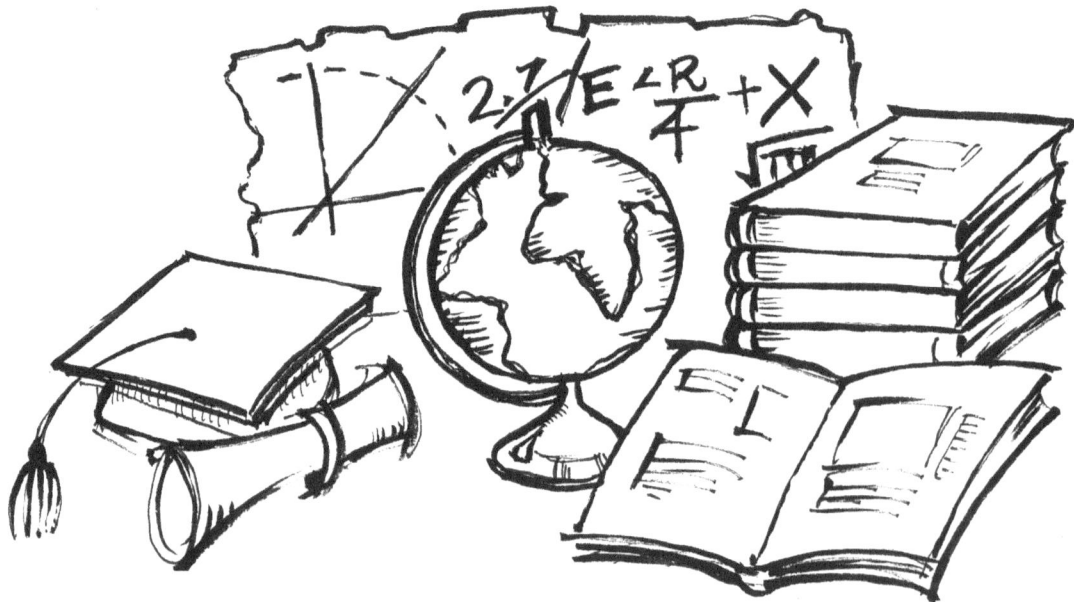

Intellectual

All growth depends upon activity. There is no development physically or intellectually without effort, and effort means work.

-Calvin Coolidge

Intellectual Dimension

Have you explored the potential benefits of maximizing your intellectual wellness? Have you considered the impact of having great problem solving and decision making skills? Do you wonder how well you have been doing in this area? I consider this "a time for growth". There is always room for growth in life and work if you are open to exploring and learning.

Ask yourself, am I doing a well as I know I can in this area? If not how is this affecting my relationship with my loved ones or co-workers? Is it affecting my ability to be more successful?

Learning stimulates growth. As you work on the intellectual dimension, you will be reminded of your capacity for growth and development. I hope that the information you are exposed to in this workbook and in your sessions with your coach will help you gain a deeper level of awareness. It is my hope that this will inspire you to make learning and growth a part of your life style choice.

In this section, I will focus on goal setting, reflection and critical thinking, because I believe that in developing competencies in these areas you will be able to set and achieve goals that will help you in all areas of your intellectual development. You will also improve your critical thinking and interpersonal intelligence.

As you begin to explore this dimension, I would like you to identify the area(s) in which you want to grow and develop.

Assessing your Intellectual Wellness

To assess your intellectual wellness, please transfer the scores from your IWQ assessment. You may want to assess different areas from the ones you assessed previously.

What areas did you assess?

_____

_____

What have you noticed about your scores?

_____

_____

What is your intellectual wellness score? _____

How long have you been scoring this number? _____

Has your life situation changed recently in any of these areas, if so which one, and how?

_____

_____

Looking ahead, what score would you like to have for intellectual wellness? _____

What makes this your ideal intellectual wellness score? _____

_____

_____

How would you like to improve your intellectual dimension?

_____

_____

How do you rate your likelihood of improving your wellness in these areas?

_____

_____

What is one thing you might need to do to get you off to a good start?

_____

_____

Goal Setting

Research has shown that those who have set, noted and shared their goals with others have far greater success than those without goals. It also shows that those who have set goals but did not write them down or communicate their goals to others are less successful. Some people believe we need goals to be happy, fulfilled and committed. I believe that goals are also important to keep us motivated and focused.

 Have you set clear, written goals for your future and made plans to accomplish them?

_____

_____

What life goal are you currently working on?

_____

_____

Why is this goal important to you and which of your values does this goal reflect?

_____

_____

It is important that your goals truly reflect your passions and values. However, if you are in a situation where you believe a particular goal is not being met, you should give yourself permission to re-establish a new goal for yourself.

There are many reasons why people set goals for themselves that do not align with their values. You may feel pressure from others such as family and friends.

For example, many people feel pressured to pursue a particular career or occupation because other family members are in that profession, or because it is highly regarded in their family and/or community. Others may feel pressured to take on a family business even when this does not reflect their true passion.

Questions

What is one passion you are currently pursuing or would like to pursue?

_____

_____

Who or what in your life helps you stay committed to your passions?

_____

_____

Goal Setting Exercise

Step1. Write down your top five goals below.

1. _____

2. _____

3. _____

4. _____

5. _____

Step 2. Read through each of your goals once.

Step 3. Restate each goal with your eyes closed and your right hand on your heart.

Step 4. Become aware of your body and senses – is there a quickening of your pulse and a tingling of excitement with any of the goals? __Yes __ No

Step 5. Notice your body's response: is there a tightening of your chest and do you feel a sense of dread about any of your goals? __Yes __ No

Step 7. Put a check mark beside the goals that resonate with your heart and excites you.

Step 8. Use the space below to make notes of how you are going to accomplish your top three goals.

One cannot successfully achieve a goal without taking risks, but it is wise to employ the five key elements of goal setting we discussed. This will ensure that you take strategic, clear and decisive actions towards reaching your goals.

Keep in mind that the thrill of reaching a goal can only be experienced by those who set them. So go ahead and overhaul your goals - I wish you much success in your goal-setting process.

Notes

_____

_____

_____

_____

Fear of Failure

Fear of failure is one reason why many people do not set goals for themselves. When we experience failure, it brings feelings of self-doubt, sadness and negative self-talk. When you encounter a challenge, it is important to acknowledge and work with your coach to set structures to support you in successfully reaching future goals. I think many people fail at achieving their goals because they have not applied one or more of the necessary key elements of strategic goal setting.

Questions

Does fear of failure prevent you from setting big goals for yourself, if so, what goal have you put off setting?

_____

_____

Do you sometimes have doubts about your ability to achieve your goals, do you still try?

_____

_____

Critical Thinking

Critical thinking allows us to think outside the box and frees us from limiting beliefs and thoughts that might otherwise hold us back.

Take the time to recognize fear, paranoia, frustration, and negative feelings within you. Recognize fear and stressful thoughts and address them quickly. When you hear the little voice of negativity in the back of your mind and ask the question: How true is this? How do I know that my thoughts are accurate?

When you begin entertaining thoughts such as
- I should not have lost my job
- why me? Why did I have to get sick?
- why is he or she picking on me?
- I don't think I can do that, or if only…

It's time to change your focus and do something different. If you focus on these thoughts, they will only serve to distract you from your true goal.

Don't make fear of failure become your focus. Take the following steps to help you conquer fear:

-Assess who you spend time with, even if they are family members
-Clean your house and clear out the dust bunnies
-Change old habits; begin a new routine or hobby
-Make new friends
-Seek out positive, motivating people in your life if you cannot afford a coach
-Challenge your thoughts with inquiry and question your thoughts
-Take new actions

Accountability

Accountability is a key factor in our ability to set and accomplish goals. Whether the goal is to learn something new, upgrade our education or to reflect on a negative trait or habit, we need to have some level of accountability to ourselves, and to one another in order to follow through.

Accountability is the act of being held responsible for our actions or inactions. It shows one's capacity to fulfill obligations in light of agreed expectations. There is a difference between responsibility and accountability; responsibility is the duty to act, while accountability is the commitment to act and be held liable. I believe that information raises awareness. When we become aware, this raises our sense of duty responsibility to do something about that which we are now aware. When we assume responsibility for something, we are now accountable to fulfilling that requirement.

To be accountable, one needs to feel valuable and significant. Working with a coach is a great way to build your confidence through acknowledgment and validation. This will help you to gradually develop your accountability muscles.

Questions

Is taking responsibility a challenge for you?

_____

_____

How comfortable are you with being accountable?

_____

_____

Would you like to work on being more responsible?

_____

_____

Problem Solving

Problem solving is a skill we each need to have in order to solve life problems. Everyone will encounter problems in their life, work or relationships. It is important to ensure that you take time to focus on what the problem is and the best possible course of action to resolve it. Keep in mind that problems are different from conflicts. While conflicts pit people against each other, problems are impersonal and require you to focus your attention on the situation. Many problems lead to conflicts because those involved fail to focus on the problem and instead lay blame and accuse others, which often results in a conflict.

Questions

How well do you handle problems?

_____

_____

Would you like to work on being a more profound problem solver?

_____

_____

Chapter Insight

As you look back on the readings and exercises in this chapter, what insights have you gained?

_____

_____

What aspects were of most importance to you?

_____

_____

Please use the chart below to note your insights, the date and your intended actions. Three months from this date, please revisit this chart to note your level of completion.

Insight/Date	Intended Action/Step	Complete 0-100%
1		
2		
3		

Reflections

What is one thing you experienced in the intellectual dimension that changed your focus or thinking?

_____

_____

How might you do things differently to change or enhance your intellectual wellness?

_____

_____

What is one personal growth area you have identified and how will it help improve your IWQ?

_____

_____

What new structures have you been able to put in place to support your personal growth?

_____

_____

Notes

_____

_____

_____

_____

All men by nature desire knowledge.

-Aristotle

A Time to be Interdependent

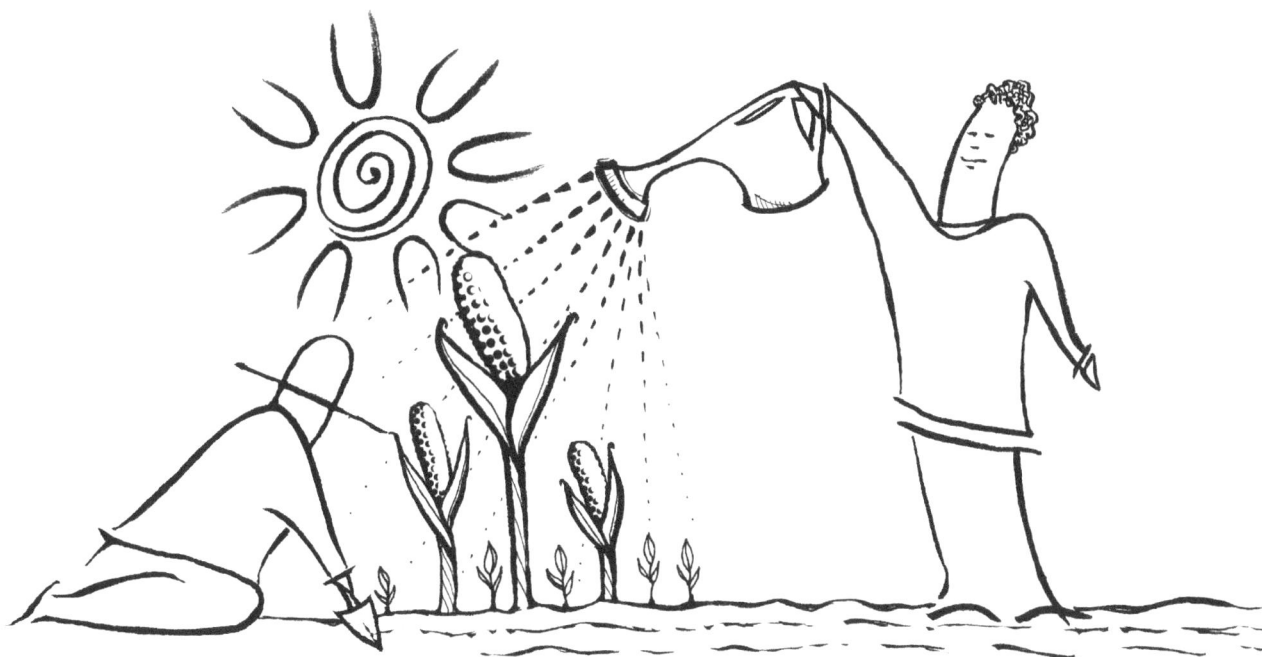

Environmental

I define comfort as self-acceptance. When we finally learn that self-care begins and ends with ourselves, we no longer demand sustenance and happiness from others.

-Jennifer Louden

Environmental Dimension

Have you experienced the benefits of being in a great environment where things are working well and others are showing respect for each and the environment? Do you wonder how well you are doing in this area? I consider this "a time to be interdependent". Life and nature reflects interdependence and sharing. We live better lives when we are in harmony with others and with our environment.

Ask yourself, am I doing a well as I know I can in this area? If not, how is this affecting my relationship with my loved ones or co-workers? Can I do something today to improve my environment? Can I do something to show more respect and understanding to others?

Our culture promotes individualism. The media and society reminds us daily of our individual rights, choices and freedoms. This is contrary to the very nature of society, where each social system is interconnected and interdependent. The current global economic crisis that has impacted every country in the world is another example of our connectedness. As you assess the environmental dimension of your life, take note of how much everything including yourself is interconnected and interdependent.

Assessing your Environmental Wellness

To assess your environmental wellness, please transfer the scores from your IWQ assessment. You may want to assess different areas from the ones you previously assessed.

What areas did you assess?

_____

_____

What have you noticed about your scores?

_____

_____

What is your environmental wellness score? _____

How long have you been scoring this number? _____

Has your life situation changed recently in any of these areas, if so which one, and how?

_____

_____

Looking ahead, what score would you like to have for environmental wellness? _____

What makes this your ideal social wellness score? _____

_____

_____

How would you like to improve your environmental dimension?

_____

_____

How do you rate your likelihood of improving your wellness in these areas?

_____

_____

What is one thing you might need to do to get you off to a good start?

_____

Personal Impact

The ability to be aware of our personal impact on others is a vital skill in maintaining a healthy interpersonal network, and in understanding the impact of our social vibrations, actions and words. When we are conscious of our impact on others and our environment, it increases our level of interpersonal intelligence, informing and equipping us to make better decisions that will improve our IWQ.

When you embark on a Personal Audit, it is important that you assess each area of your life. You will notice that there will be some areas in your life that are working quite well. Please take time to acknowledge your efforts in these areas; everyone has areas of excellence and you do too. Your acknowledgement of this is important in cementing the awareness of your current capacity, and will be the benchmark from which you will improve other areas that are not working as well. Such an audit helps you to uncover deficits or unintended contributions to your own wellness that may be negatively impacting your relationships. This heightened awareness will serve to increase your sense of responsibility and motivate you to make positive improvements.

Though we are led to believe that our actions and choices are independent, in an audit, it quickly becomes apparent that the chain of events resulting from a person's actions can have lasting and at times devastating consequences for the larger community. For example, the individual who discards a lighted cigarette butt in the forest can cause a wildfire, destroying dozens of homes and risking many lives in the community. Don't go through life with unintended consequences. Take time to learn what actions and consequences make your life healthy and positive.

Questions

Is there an action you take that is having unintended consequence on your relationship?

_____

_____

Is there an action that someone in your network is taking that is negatively impacting you?

_____

If we are able to identify our contributions to the challenges we face, we will spend less energy projecting blame and anger onto those we believe responsible for those issues. We will then ask the question, why am I harbouring resentment, and what do I believe about this situation that makes it so painful and difficult to repair? As we ask these questions, we may discover underlying beliefs that may help us see our contributions to the situation. By doing this, we can take corrective actions to repair relationships, become socially conscious, give back to society or take steps to become socially responsible, and improve our IWQ.

Social Responsibility

Each of us has a social responsibility to contribute to the wellness of ourselves and to others in our family or social network. It is our responsibility to obey the laws and be respectful of others' rights and diverse needs. When we fail to do this or are negatively engaged in conflicting habits or actions, we detract from our own wellness and neglect our social responsibility.

Those who choose to harass or bully others, act in a racist, sexist or prejudiced way, display poor social consciousness and disharmony with their environment. These actions show that they shirk their responsibility to respect diversity, which is a requirement for living in harmony with our environment, each other and the universe.

Every workplace has a legal and social responsibility to see to the overall Interpersonal Wellness of their employees. In a similar way, each individual has a moral responsibility to positively contribute to the wellness of their relationships at work and at home. Those who maintain excellent relationships at work, and have poor family relationships with their children or spouse at home are failing to observe the interdependence of life and relationships.

When we invest in all our interpersonal relationships, we reap positive benefits in all areas of our lives including in the form of healthy interactions. Individuals who have developed a high level of Interpersonal Wellness skills and competencies will experience increased success, productivity and effectiveness in all areas of life. They will also have higher IWQ, enjoy collaborative working relationships and will radiate positive social vibrations that will improve morale and vitality.

Questions

Can your actions be considered socially responsible?

Is there a work or personal relationship that fosters your sense of social responsibility?

_____

_____

What situations or atmosphere make it difficult for you to be socially responsible?

_____

_____

Healthy Living Environment

What is a healthy living environment? A healthy living environment is one in which care is taken to ensure that the inhabitants do not suffer any harm from their surroundings. This may include the physical surrounding such as the cleanliness of the area, personal safety, and adequate protection from pests, debris and physical harm. It also includes the social and emotional health of your environment such as positive contacts, optimism, low rate of stress, and the absence of mental or physically abuse.   It should also be free of harassment, racism, discrimination and stereotypes as these are great causes of social isolation and stress.

Questions

Do you live or work in an environment that is harmful to your health?

_____

_____

Is there an action you are taking that may cause undue stress for others?

_____

_____

Chapter Insight

As you look back on the readings and exercises in this chapter, what insights have you gained?

_____

_____

What aspects were of most importance to you?

_____

_____

What new skill or competencies will you need to learn or develop?

_____

_____

Please use the chart below to note your insights, the date and your intended actions. Three months from this date, please revisit this chart to note your level of completion.

Insight/Date	Intended Action/Step	Complete 0-100%
1		
2		
3		

Reflections

What is one thing you experienced in the environmental dimension that changed your focus or thinking about respect and interdependence?

_____

_____

How might you do things differently to change or enhance your social consciousness?

_____

_____

What is one personal growth area you have identified and how will it help improve your sense of social responsibility?

_____

_____

What new structures will you need to put in place to support your growth in this area?

_____

_____

Notes

_____

_____

_____

_____

In all things of nature there is something of the marvelous.

- Aristotle

A Time to Plan

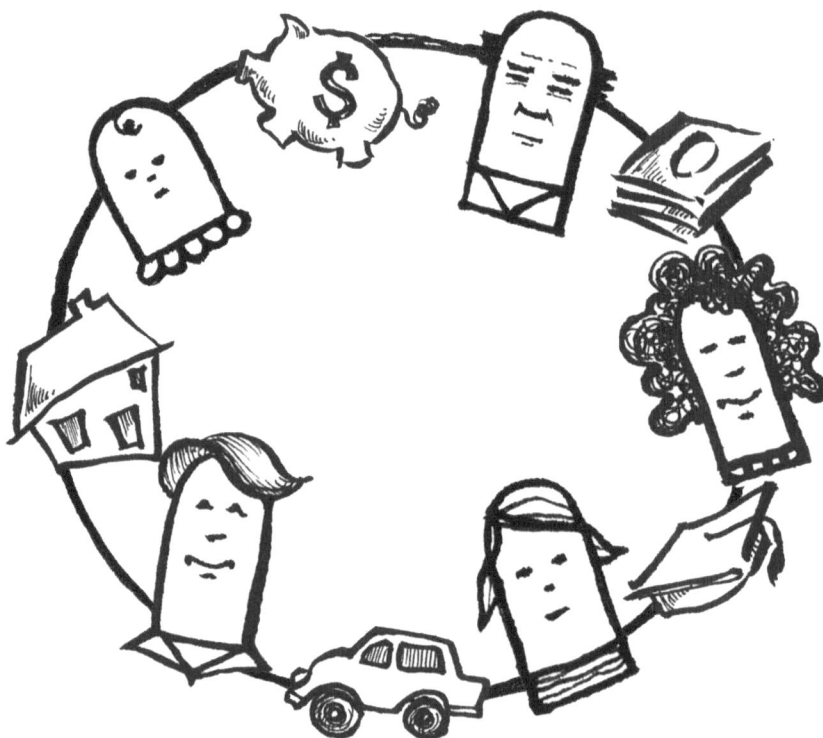

Financial

Poor is the man who does not know his own intrinsic worth and tends to measure everything by relative value. A man of financial wealth who values himself by his financial net worth is poorer than a poor man who values himself by his intrinsic self worth.

- Sidney Madwed

Financial Dimension

Have you explored the potential benefits of having great financial freedom and success? Do you wonder how your life would be different? What would you do with all the extra time? Well this is a time to assess how well you are doing in this area. I consider this "a time to plan". No matter what your financial state, others have been there and turned it around and so can you.

Ask yourself, am I doing a well as I know I can in this area? If not how is this affecting my relationship with my loved ones and my life? How is this affecting my success and my future happiness?

I would like to challenge your views about financial worth. Many individuals have limiting beliefs about their earning potential or capacity to own great wealth. Many religions teach that those who are poor are also blessed. As a result, many cultural norms convey disdain for the accumulation and possession of great wealth. This often leads to conflicting money management beliefs and actions. People often face challenging feelings such as anxiety, guilt and disappointments about wanting and having money, which can negatively impact the financial well-being of many.

As you work through the financial dimension, I would like you to pay close attention to your beliefs about money. Note the thoughts you have about your capacity to earn or possess more money. Note your feelings about having a rich and abundant life, and take the time to direct your focus onto what you want to have in your life as you apply prayer, meditation, visualization or any of the strategies we discussed earlier.

Many believe that by being grateful for your current financial reality you will open up new channels for financial blessings you had not imagined possible. Some also believe that we are not all rich because we are not all prepared to handle more money responsibly. There are many schools of thought on money acquisition and management, so I won't do that here. However, in his book, *The Science of Getting Rich*, Wallace D. Wattles, claims that it's normal for each of us to want to be rich, as this is a way to living a more expressive and abundant life. He advocates the belief that by being rich we can live a rewarding life and can be of more value to the world. There are many other books and resources on finances, getting rich, managing money and budgeting that may be valuable for you. I encourage you to read more on the subject.

Assessing your Financial Wellness

To assess your financial wellness, please transfer the scores from your IWQ assessment. You may want to assess different areas from the ones you previously assessed.

What areas did you assess?

_____

_____

What have you noticed about your scores?

_____

_____

What is your financial wellness score? _____

How long have you been scoring this number? _____

Has your life situation changed recently in any of these areas, if so which one, and how?

_____

_____

Looking ahead, what score would you like to have for financial wellness? _____

What makes this your ideal financial wellness score?

_____

_____

_____

How would you like to improve your financial dimension, in what area and by what action?

_____

Do you experience feelings of doubt about having more money, or are you hopeful and thankful for what you have and what you can do with it?

_____

_____

How do you rate your likelihood of improving your wellness in this dimension?

_____

_____

What is one thing you might need to do to get you off to a good start?

_____

_____

Interdependence

Often, when we ask for financial solutions we are told to make a budget and stick to it. There are times when it's important to stop and pay attention to the realities of our income and expenses. However, it is also important to examine limiting beliefs you hold about money.

Our financial reality can often reflect deficits in other areas of our lives that we first need to acknowledge and manage in order to become successful at reaching our financial goals.

Financial health does not correlate with one's occupation or earnings. There are individuals who are financially well who have earned meagre incomes all their lives. There are also those who have had substantial earnings, yet their financial reserve is nil. Keep this in mind when next you differentiate your necessities from the things you want.

When we embrace negative thoughts about our lack of financial wealth, we feel dejected, low energy, and deflated. This arouses a negative self-image and pessimism that causes us to focus on our lack rather than give thanks for what we have. This can potentially have a negative impact in all other areas of our lives, creating stress, anger, frustration, illnesses and interpersonal conflicts. When you receive thoughts of your lack, chase them away with thought of gratitude for what you have. As a result, you will send out positive social vibrations that will transmit positive feelings to those in your social network.

Questions

Do you hold negative thoughts about your financial wellness?

_____

_____

What beliefs do you hold about your ability to improve your financial wellness?

_____

_____

When we define ourselves by the amount of money in our bank account and use that as a measurement of self-worth, we do ourselves a disservice.

We may need to change our thoughts and beliefs about money in order to begin viewing money the way it is meant to be. Money is designed to one currency of exchange, as we will discuss later, there are several currencies of exchange that you can access.

The Bible states, *"For the love of money is the root of all kinds of evil. And some people, craving money, have wandered from the true faith and pierced themselves with many sorrows."* 1 Timothy 6:10 (NLT).

The above text is a metaphor or parable which demonstrates that using money well does not require us to have a devotion to it; rather, financial wellness requires us to exercise good judgment in the use and management of the money we have acquired.

Questions

What's your view of having more money?

_____

_____

Do you have a passion for money or for the things money can buy?

_____

_____

What is one way you could contribute to the world if you had more money?

_____

_____

Do you believe that the money coming your way is a gift to be used with care?

_____

_____

Money and Stress

When we are stressed about our lack of money this can be very distracting. It robs us of our ability to be conscious; we lack the presence of mind and exuberance we could otherwise have and we become fixated on our money or lack thereof.

These thoughts rob us of time to grow spiritually. They negatively impact our self-esteem. Many of us hold the belief that how much money we have defines us and our identity. In those case, the shame that accompanies not having money impacts us emotionally and is often manifested as stress, anger, resentment and envy.

These feelings negatively impact our ability to interact with others in a healthy way. We become much angrier at work and have less patience with clients and customers and we become easily irritated and agitated.

The IWS model views the individual as an interconnected interpersonal network and highlights how each part of life interrelates. When we are connected with each other, we feel a sense of belonging and acceptance. This is supposed to support us through the tough and challenging times of life. We often hear stories of how happy poor people are and how simple their lives are. Could it be that we have it all wrong and that money might just make our lives more complicated?

Since many people identify themselves by their occupations, this determines their financial status. By solely identifying yourself this way, you become automatically associated with a certain life-style and the related stresses that come with maintaining it. This is when we begin to miss the simple life.

Questions

From where do you draw your self-worth?

_____

_____

What related financial stress comes from maintaining your current life-style?

_____

_____

Money Management

"I can buy what I want, it's my money!" I think we all feel this way from time to time, but the drawback of this is that if we don't always have the cash to pay now, we put it on credit and end up paying twice as much, or more later as interest payments.

Many of us lack the skill of proper money management, so we end up spending more than we earn, buying on credit and carrying a huge debt load. Often we become so ensnared by passing fads or fashion that we feel obliged to make unnecessary purchases and get stuck making payments later. Since we did not have the money in the first place, we end up not having the money to make the payments later and so the vicious cycle of living on credit begins.

Good money management skills begin with your having a clear idea of your income and expenses, tracking where you are currently spending your money, and assessing whether you are happy with what you are spending your money on. If you are not sure where it's being spent, then you need to track your dollars and come up with a plan on where to spend your money and stick with it.

Questions:

Are you happy with how your money is being spent?

_____

Are you aware of your spending habits?

_____

_____

Are you finding it hard to pay all the bills on time?

_____

_____

Is there a danger that your money management strategies are getting you further in debt?

_____

_____

Savings

How would your life be different in you began saving some money each week? It does not have to be a lot, it could be just ten dollars of even five dollars more a week. This could add up to hundreds of dollars over the years. Too often we think that a dime is too little to save and we walk away leaving a penny on the counter and not collecting our spare change. Have you ever considered that if you leave a penny on the counter five hundred times in your life that would add up to $5.00? What if you did that a thousand times – this would add up to $10.00. Ask yourself, if you were to put away $10.00 a week over 30 years how much would you have saved? What if you could do more than that and put away a bit more by cutting out one restaurant meal per week? You would see your net worth begin to grow and you would begin to feel richer.

Studies have shown it is wise for us to save at least 10% of our income. Now wouldn't that change your reality? Go ahead give it a try and begin saving something this week and don't stop no matter the temptation to purchase something becomes.

Questions:

Would it be difficult to put a small amount of money away each week?

_____

_____

If you had to choose a way to save, what would be the most effective means you could begin in the next week?

_____

_____

Financial Equity

Everyone has equity or worth. It is true though that many of us go through life without ever becoming aware of our worth. We often think of equity as money in the bank or value in property but that is not all true. Money is only one currency of life. There other forms of currency. One such currency is barter. We can learn to utilize our equity in many ways to raise capital or to exchange our services. Have you ever considered what you may be able to trade or barter with (beside body parts)?

The equity you barter with may be a service, an idea, a skill you may have or a resource you have developed to solve a problem in the world or in your community. We each need to learn to view our financial equity differently from what is on the balance sheet. Too often I see people beating up on themselves because society has dictated that their equity is nil. It's time to take your power back and view your equity as part of your own unique genius that can be exchanged for another service of for cash.

Questions:

Can you think of a service of skill that you can exchange as a means towards increasing your financial equity?

_____

_____

What is one skill that you can legally trade for a fee or for other none monetary means?

_____

Who might be most likely to engage or exchange services with you and why?

_____

_____

Chapter Insight

As you look back on the readings and exercises in this chapter, what insights have you gained?

_____

_____

What aspects were of most importance to you?

_____

_____

Please use the chart below to note your insights, the date and your intended actions. Three months from this date, please revisit this chart to note your level of completion.

Insight/Date	Intended Action/Step	Complete 0-100%
1		
2		
3		

Reflections

What is one thing you experienced in the financial dimension that changed your focus or thinking?

_____

_____

How might you do things differently to change or enhance your financial wellness?

_____

_____

What is one area of you have identified and how will it help improve your financial wellness?

_____

_____

What new structures have you been able to put in place to support your personal growth?

_____

_____

Notes:

_____

_____

_____

_____

In the arena of human life the honors and rewards fall to those who show their good qualities.

-Aristotle

A Time to Be Vibrant

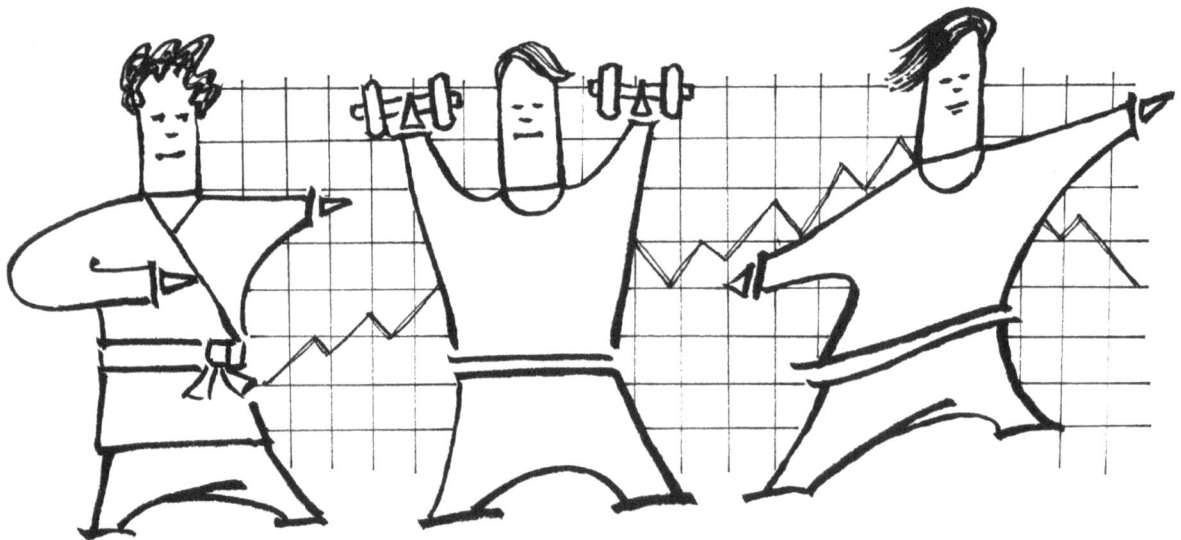

Physical

He who has health has hope; and he who has hope has everything.

~Arabic Proverb

Physical Dimension

Have you explored the potential benefits of having great physical health and wellness? Do you know how well you are doing in this area? Do you have the energy you need to complete your days work? Are you unable to concentrate and interact with loved ones? Ask yourself, how is this impacting your relationships? It is never too late to change your physical wellness by changing unhealthy habits and forming new freeing ones. I consider this "a time to be vibrant". It is a time to take action, to get moving and to impact your physical and personal wellness.

Do you have loved ones who are concerned about the state of your health and wellness? What can you do to relieve their worries? How might you express your gratitude and appreciation to them?

Ask yourself, am I doing a well as I know I can in this area? If not how is this affecting my relationship with my loved ones, my life or career? How is this impacting how I am experiencing my life now and how well I will experience my life in my golden years? Are there actions I can take now to invest in my future health or to turn my health around?

Many people associate the term wellness with something physical. I believe wellness is a state of being and thinking that is reflected in all the dimensions in your life.

There are things you can physically do to maintain your health and wellness and they include taking care to eat well by maintaining a diet that is nutritious, by getting proper rest, by taking time each day to build your muscles through some form of exercise and by taking care of your health and ensuring that you limit unhealthy substances and addictive foods and drugs. It is your responsibility to take care of your physical health and wellness as this will ultimately impact your wellness in all the other dimensions.

To deny this responsibility is to flirt with disaster. Each one of us has a duty to learn about our body and its overall care.

Assessing your Physical Wellness

To assess your physical wellness, please transfer the scores from your IWQ assessment. You may want to assess different areas from the ones you previously assessed.

What areas did you assess?

_____

_____

What have you noticed about your scores?

_____

_____

What is your physical wellness score? _____

How long have you been scoring this number? _____

Has your life situation changed recently in any of these areas, if so which one, and how?

_____

_____

Looking ahead, what score would you like to have in physical wellness? _____

What makes this your ideal physical wellness score? _____

_____

_____

How would you like to improve your physical dimension?

_____

_____

How do you rate your likelihood of improving your wellness habits?

_____

_____

What is one thing you might need to do to get you off to a good start?

_____

_____

Affirmations

Affirmation is an effective strategy that can aid you in developing a positive outlook and build-up your self esteem. For example, Jane gives herself positive affirmations daily by writing in her journal every morning about the things she did well the day before and her goals for the next day.

In this section, I would like to invite you to make some personal affirmations to keep yourself motivated to complete the necessary changes in your life. Positive affirmations can help you to move forward and squelch negative self-talk.

As you become more aware of your personal responsibilities to maintain a healthy balance in each area of your life, take this time to begin affirming yourself. The following are example of affirmations that you can utilize:

Positive Affirmations

Today I can make a difference.

Today I can begin to recreate my future.

I have the ability to become the person I want to be.

I can take one action today towards becoming the new me.

I have personal worth and great attributes to give to the world.

I don't have to be nudged, coerced or prompted to do the things that have been a struggle for me in the past, because I am my new self.

Questions:

Do you positively affirm yourself daily? How do you affirm yourself?

_____

_____

What changes occur in your day when you affirm yourself or another person?

_____

_____

Take some time and write out some positive affirmations that are reflective of your needs in the space below:

Personal Affirmations

1._____

2._____

3._____

4._____

5._____

Power of Beliefs

Our lives and expectations are based solely on our beliefs. Sometimes we hold beliefs that defy logic; for example, I may believe that I can eat as many calories as I want and still attain my weight loss goal. This is however, not logical. What we believe about something does not change basic life principles. By holding onto those beliefs we deny that certain life principles apply to us, and by failing to observe these life principles, we soon discover that the consequences do indeed relate to us.

Questions:

What beliefs do you adopt about your physical wellness?

_____

_____

How might these beliefs be contributing to your current physical challenges?

_____

_____

What new thought can you hold in the next seven days that will get you closer to changing those beliefs?

_____

_____

Is there a time when these beliefs served you well?

_____

_____

What beliefs do you hold that are supporting you positively?

_____

_____

Physical Interdependence

Our physical appearance often reflects our level of wellness in the other areas of our lives. It will reflect things such as high stress, our stamina and energy level, strength, proper nutrition, and getting adequate rest. I believe that our physical appearance is the most revealing factor in the level of wellness we are experiencing in the other dimensions of our lives. A make-over of our appearance is much more than weight loss through diet and exercise, or by refreshing our wardrobe. It instead requires us to do a wellness audit of all the dimensions of our lives to ensure that we are living as best as we can in each area.

Research has shown a relationship between our diet, exercise and adequate rest on the overall quality of our physical health. Self-care is no longer optional, but rather a personal obligation we have to ourselves and to our relationships.

When we practice proper self-care, we feel great and have better mental energy, a healthier outlook on life and more stamina. We are better able to focus and gain clarity on our goals and the actions required to get us there; and we are also better able to communicate and interact well in our relationships.

Questions

What does your physical appearance reveal about you?

_____

_____

What can you do to change, improve or maintain your physical appearance?

_____

_____

Chronic Disease

There is new research citing that the some chronic diseases may have to do with pre-birth issues with our parents or environments in developmental years and some are linked to traumas in our early childhood. Regardless of the risks involved it is also proven that we can defer or reduce our chances to get some if not all of these diseases with diet and exercise programs, as well as by managing our stress level to just a healthy amount of stress.

We are in essence what we eat and what we think. Every thought we have triggers a physiological response whether we are aware of it or not. This means that we should try our best to ensure that our thoughts are stress free at least a quarter of the time. This will go a long way towards shielding us from hereditary chronic and other life style generated chronic diseases.

If you already have chronic illnesses you can do things like a change of diet and exercise to minimize the risk of them getting worst or to help manage them.

Chapter Insight

As you look back on the readings and exercises in this chapter, what insights have you gained?

_____

_____

What aspects were of most importance to you?

_____

_____

Please use the chart below to note your insights, the date and your intended actions. Three months from this date, please revisit this chart to note your level of completion.

Insight/Date	Intended Action/Step	Complete 0-100%
1		
2		
3		

Reflections

What is one thing you experienced in the physical dimension that changed your focus or thinking?

_____

How might you do things differently to change or enhance your physical wellness?

_____

_____

What is one action you can take, and how will it help improve your physical wellness or health?

_____

_____

List three people who are available to support your wellness journey?

_____

_____

What is one thing you have done in the past that has helped you improve your personal wellness?

_____

_____

Notes:

_____

_____

_____

_____

It is the nature of desire not to be satisfied, and most men live only for the gratification of it.

-Aristotle

A Time to Experience Your Best Self

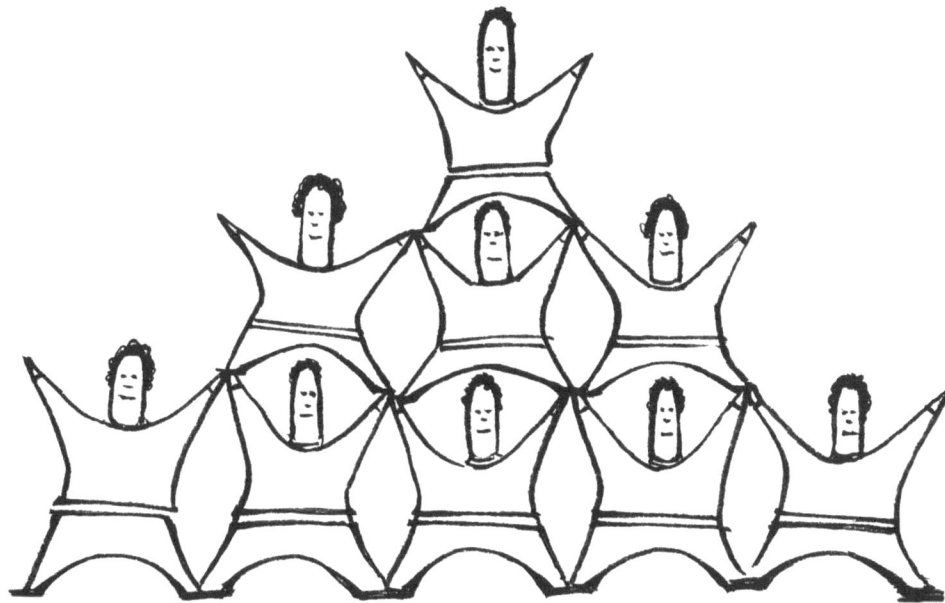

Interpersonal

Your most precious possession is not your financial assets. Your most precious possession is the people you have working there, and what they carry around in their heads, and their ability to work together.

-Robert Reich

Interpersonal Dimension

Have you explored the potential benefits of having great relationships and the life that you want? Do you wonder how well others are experiencing you in your personal or professional network? I consider this "a time to experience your best self". This means that it is never too late to change how others will experience you in the future. You can do this by managing your wellness in the other eight areas of the Interpersonal Wellness System model.

Ask yourself, how well am I experiencing my relationships? How is this relationship affecting my loved ones or co-workers? How can I invest in my relationships now for the future?

I believe that the real meaning of life is going to be assessed by the relationships we have developed and fostered in this life-time. Having measured your personal wellness in each dimension, and tallied a score that revealed your overall wellness in that area; the question is: so what? I would like to respond in this section of the workbook and give you an opportunity to put it all together. When we add eight scores and divide the sum by eight we get your IWQ. This reflects the overall wellness in all areas of your life at this time, informing you of your capacity to contribute to the wellness of your life and relationships.

Of course this is not a permanent state but the most current state from which you can decide to make necessary changes. The message here is that when we maintain optimal wellness in all areas of our lives, we increase our capacity to contribute optimally to our interpersonal relationships. As a result these relationships will flourish and become rich and rewarding; giving back to us positive vibrations in the form of collaboration, esteem, fun, power to conquer life challenges, and a sense of belonging. Such relationships become our foundation and interpersonal wellness bank accounts in which we invest and gain dividends in the form of positive interactions.

Interpersonal Relationship Audit

Now that you have completed your IWQ assessment you can assess a relationship of your choice. Please pick a relationship of your choice below:

1. Parent/Guardian
2. Sibling/Child
3. Supervisor/Manager/Team leader
4. Spouse/Partner
5. Neighbour/Community/Church

As you complete this section of the workbook, take some time to reflect on the relationship you want to have and the steps you can take to create that experience.

Please answer the following questions about your relationship, using the same scale of 1 – 10, on which 1 is poor and 10 is excellent, to measure the level of wellness in your relationship. Upon completion, add your numbers and divide (÷) them by 12 which signifies the number of questions in the exercise.

1. How would you rate your relationship with yourself, and with the other person(s) in this relationship? _____
2. How would you rate your ability to manage conflict in this relationship? _____
3. How would you rate the level of positive social vibrations that is felt in this relationship? _____
4. How would you rate the level of encouragement and personal power you draw from this relationship? _____
5. How would you rate the level of support, assistance, team work and collaboration you bring to this relationship? _____
6. How would you rate the level of support, assistance, team work and collaboration you receive in this relationship? _____
7. How would you rate your ability to fit in or your sense of belonging in this relationship? _____
8. How would you rate your regard for and admiration of the other person(s) in this relationship? _____
9. How would you rate the level of respect and good opinion others in this relationship have of you? _____
10. How would you rate your influence in this relationship? _____
11. How would you rate the level of fun in this relationship? _____
12. How would you rate the level of influence others in this relationship have on you? _____

As you complete these questions, think of things you can do to begin contributing more or differently to the relationship(s) that you have assessed.

Knowing your IWQ is to know what you have to offer to the world-a place where relationships matter.

Interpersonal Relationship Wellness

Reflect on the rating you have given to these areas in your life as you answer the questions below.

What have you noticed about the way you rated your relationship?

_____

_____

What is your overall relationship score? _____

How long have you been scoring this number? _____

Has your life situation or relationship changed recently? If so, how?

_____

_____

Looking ahead, at what level would you like this relationship to be scored? _____

Why would this be an ideal score? _____

_____

_____

How would you like to improve your relationship?

_____

_____

When was a time that your relationship worked well?

_____

_____

What things, place or people have a positive influence on your relationship wellness?

_____

_____

What is one thing you might need to do to get you off to a good start?

_____

_____

Relationship Meaning

The IWS model shows that we derive meaning from communication and interaction with each other by sending out social vibrations to those in our social or interpersonal networks. From this they derive meaning, constructed from the energy or social vibrations we emit, through our interactions with others. This is often referred to as 'morale' in groups or 'bad vibes' in individuals. As we cannot touch or see these, I refer to them as social vibrations.

Since we have not been able to measure, see or touch the social vibrations of a group, team, relationship or person, we have thus far referred to this energy as morale or vibes. If it's negative we have used terms such as unpleasant, low morale, bad vibes and toxic. I hope that the IWQ will help to broaden the discourse in this area, allowing for a more descriptive term to refer to social vibrations. It is my hope that from this measurement we can glean information as to how low, how high, how well and where we need to do work, grow and improve our IWQ; and by so doing, our interactions with others.

We can infect, contaminate, attract or detract from our interpersonal relationships. We have the ability to manage our social vibrations by taking care of our wellness in the dimensions presented in the IWS model.

If we regularly audit each of our life dimensions, we will be able to make positive contributions to our relationships by making small changes in our self. In return, we will make interpersonal investments governed by a system of interdependence that can only be negatively affected if we stop assuming our personal responsibility to manage our own wellness.

Questions

What kinds of social vibrations are you sending out to your interpersonal network?

_____

_____

Are you aware of how your social vibrations impact those around you?

_____

_____

What is one area you will need to work on to maintain your Interpersonal Wellness?

_____

_____

What is one thing in your life that helps you to contribute positively to your interpersonal relationships?

_____

_____

What one area of your life do you think, if addressed, will have a positive impact on your relationships and in return, your IWQ?

_____

_____

Interpersonal Conflicts

Often we are unable to progress or improve an interpersonal relationship because we are embroiled in conflict. Conflict is a reality in any relationship. The challenge is in the way we choose to respond to the conflict, as this will determine whether the conflict progresses to become a negative conflict or is seen as an opportunity to change and grow the relationship.

In this section, I want to alert you to the different conflict phases and suggest how you can assess whether your conflict situation is in any of the three phases discussed more fully in my book *Getting Ready For Mediation: A Pre-Mediation Concept.* To do this, let's look at the conflict progression phases.

Conflict Progression Phases

The three conflict progression phases I have identified are Conceptual, Central and Protracted. A conflict will manifest differently in each phase; this is why it's important to know what phase your conflict is in, to determine what actions will be required as appropriate resolution options.

Conceptual Phase

This is the first phase of a conflict and it is usually characterized by feelings of frustration, anger, suspicion, blaming, and other unproductive emotional reactions. At this early stage, the conflict involves one or two parties. The chart on the next page will show what to look for and a range of resolution options for this phase.

Central Phase

This is the second phase of a conflict where alignment and coalition takes place. This means that each person in the conflict will seek to share their frustrations and confusion about the conflict and seek out others who share and support their views. This can also be termed as gathering allies to support their argument or side of the conflict. At this time, the conflict has a greater likelihood of further escalation if not resolved soon.

The escalation and intervention options are indicated in the conflict progression table below

Conflict Phase	Emotions	Escalation	Intervention

Conceptual	Anger Anxiety Doubt Fear	Suspicion Distrust Miscommunication	Individual development Awareness Raising Anger-management Coaching
Central	Resentment Frustration	Alignment Gossip Sabotage	Group intervention Mediation Group coaching
Protracted	Dislike Hate	Antagonizing Competition Disrespect Dissention Threat Violence	Group intervention Training Group coaching Culture redesign

Protracted Phase

This is the third stage of the conflict progression cycle. It is where the conflict takes on a protracted or entrenched state. In this phase, all activities and communications are done in opposition to the other party. The actions as you will see on the chart below will be conflict ridden and destructive, creating a culture of competition. In this phase, the parties in conflict are consumed by the dynamics and their actions and treatment of each other is often destructive, unproductive, detrimental and costly. At this point, most behaviours and actions are aimed at destroying, retaliating, or threatening the opposing side.

The following chart outlines the three phases of conflict progression and depicts the escalation of conflict and the role that emotions play in conflict escalation and progression.

Questions

Are you currently experiencing any of the above in one of your interpersonal relationships?

_____

_____

What helps you to address the issues in your life to prevent conflict escalation?

_____

_____

If your current conflict situation in your relationship is to be resolved, what would that require of you?

_____

_____

Conflict Life Cycle

Research on this topic has revealed that the rate at which conflict progresses from phase to phase depends upon a number of factors. I know that while some conflicts progress slowly, others move quite rapidly through the phases. Some conflicts may skip an entire phase, while others are enmeshed in the phases, showing characteristics of all. As a result, it may be difficult to depict a particular dimension that fits a conflict situation, at which time I believe the resolution options need to be very strategically determined and a third party conflict coach or mediator is to be brought in. The following are some factors that greatly influence this progression:

- The persons involved
- The disputing issues
- The environment
- The level of alignment and its influences
- The parties' desire for resolution

As you think of the conflict progression phases and the conflict life cycle, think of a conflict situation in your relationship and how it progress, then take some time to set goals for your relationship that also includes how you will assess and resolve future conflicts.

Interpersonal Success Goals

As I mentioned in the goal-setting section in the previous chapter, we all need goals to motivate and stimulate us. Take time to set some relationship goals for yourself.

Goals

List five goals you would like to accomplish in the next 90 days in the relationship of your choice.

Goal 1 _____

Goal 2 _____

Goal 3 _____

Goal 4 _____

Goal 5 _____

Conflict Progression Exercise

Based on the phases of conflict progression discussed, briefly describe a conflict phase that you are experiencing or have experienced.

_____

_____

If you are currently experiencing a conflict situation, describe the characteristics of the conflict at this time.

_____

_____

Can you describe how this conflict progressed through the phases? Please clearly describe your responses, actions, and attitudes?

_____

Looking back, is there anything you would change?

What have you learned about yourself or the other person(s) involved in this conflict?

What beliefs do you hold about yourself, the other person, or the situation that you are now able to view differently?

What is one action you are taking in a conflict situation that you would like to change?

How might you go about changing that and what would be difficult about doing so?

Conclusion

I want to encourage you to continue to assess all the areas of your life to maintain what you have worked so hard to achieve. I believe that our greatest purpose on this planet is to develop and maintain healthy interpersonal relationships, in order to experience our best self.   Each area is valuable and contributes equally to our total wellness and to the wellness of our relationships.

Because we are a system of interdependent parts, your wellness in each of the eight areas will determine your IWQ – your capacity to contribute to the wellness of the interpersonal relationships in your life. Remember that these relationships give back to you in the form of collaboration, belonging and esteem, which often surpasses your contribution, allowing you to reap dividends in the form of successful relationships that are fulfilling and rewarding.

As noted in the Introduction, because Jack's IWQ is 4.75, he could only contribute up to 4.75 to his life and relationships. Our energy, attitude, thoughts and vibrations are part of what we bring to our relationships at work or at home. If we are in an unhealthy personal or workplace relationship, and fail to maintain our wellness, we should not expect to have a perfect life. It just doesn't work that way.

So, if you are physically unwell, or are having emotional challenges, you may find yourself snapping at clients, or being rude to your employees or co-workers. If this is the case, you are not being conscious or efficient in building healthy workplace relationships.

Whenever there is a deficit in any of the eight dimension of your life, inevitably it will impact on your interpersonal network and on the health and wellness of the other areas. So, I urge you to do your Personal Wellness audit every six months to ensure that you remain in control of your life and what you contribute to your relationship and your success.

Chapter Insight

As you look back on the readings and exercises in this chapter, what insights have you gained?

_____

_____

What aspects were of most importance to you?

_____

_____

 Please use the chart below to note your insights, the date and your intended actions. Three months from this date, please revisit this chart to note your level of completion.

Insight/Date	Intended Action/Step	Complete 0-100%

1		
2		
3		

Reflections

What is one thing you experienced in the interpersonal dimension that changed your focus or thinking?

_____

_____

How might you do things differently to change or enhance your interpersonal wellness?

_____

_____

What is one personal growth area you have identified and how will it help improve your IWQ?

_____

_____

What new structures have you been able to put in place to support your interpersonal wellness growth?

_____

The universe requires all of us to contribute and to create something. Everything we do has a consequence. Therefore, when we cease to create, we are, in essence, denying who we are and what we are meant to do and be. By doing, we become. By assessing your IWQ, you will be able to see whether or not you are utilizing your capacity to create the kinds of interpersonal relationships you are capable of having.

Take some time to redo your IWQ on the next page to see what changes have occurred for you. I wish you much success!

For the things we have to learn before we can do them, we learn by doing them.

-Aristotle

Interpersonal Wellness System Model

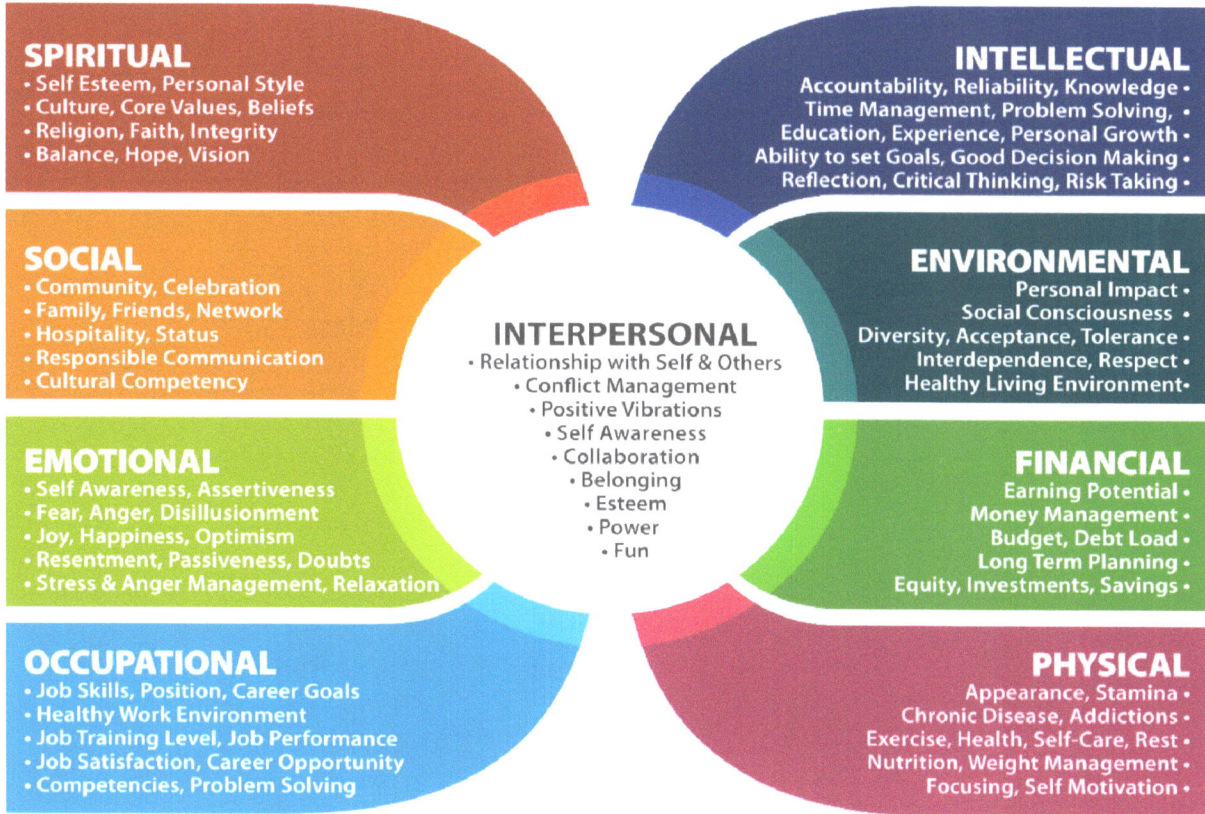

SPIRITUAL
- Self Esteem, Personal Style
- Culture, Core Values, Beliefs
- Religion, Faith, Integrity
- Balance, Hope, Vision

INTELLECTUAL
- Accountability, Reliability, Knowledge
- Time Management, Problem Solving,
- Education, Experience, Personal Growth
- Ability to set Goals, Good Decision Making
- Reflection, Critical Thinking, Risk Taking

SOCIAL
- Community, Celebration
- Family, Friends, Network
- Hospitality, Status
- Responsible Communication
- Cultural Competency

ENVIRONMENTAL
- Personal Impact
- Social Consciousness
- Diversity, Acceptance, Tolerance
- Interdependence, Respect
- Healthy Living Environment

INTERPERSONAL
- Relationship with Self & Others
- Conflict Management
- Positive Vibrations
- Self Awareness
- Collaboration
- Belonging
- Esteem
- Power
- Fun

EMOTIONAL
- Self Awareness, Assertiveness
- Fear, Anger, Disillusionment
- Joy, Happiness, Optimism
- Resentment, Passiveness, Doubts
- Stress & Anger Management, Relaxation

FINANCIAL
- Earning Potential
- Money Management
- Budget, Debt Load
- Long Term Planning
- Equity, Investments, Savings

OCCUPATIONAL
- Job Skills, Position, Career Goals
- Healthy Work Environment
- Job Training Level, Job Performance
- Job Satisfaction, Career Opportunity
- Competencies, Problem Solving

PHYSICAL
- Appearance, Stamina
- Chronic Disease, Addictions
- Exercise, Health, Self-Care, Rest
- Nutrition, Weight Management
- Focusing, Self Motivation

® Joyce Odidison

Interpersonal Wellness Quotient

Spiritual	Social	Emotional	Occupational	Intellectual	Environmental	Financial	Physical
Total =	Total =	Total =	Total =	Total =	Total =	Total =	Total =
Total ÷ 5 =	Total ÷ 5 =	Total ÷ 5 =	Total ÷ 5 =	Total ÷ 5 =	Total ÷ 5 =	Total ÷ 5 =	Total ÷ 5 =

(Add all 8 totals and divide the sum by 8 to get your IWQ) Total= _____ ÷ 8 = _____

Notes:

_____

_____

_____

_____

_____

_____

_____

_____

_____

_____

_____

_____

_____

_____

_____

_____

_____

_____

_____

_____

_____

_____

References

Attwood, J. B. and Chris. 2008. *The Passion Test The Effortless Path to Discovering Your Life Purpose*. Penguin Group Publishing.

Beck, Judith. S. 1995. *Cognitive Therapy. The Guilford Press*.

Bishop, A. 2005. *Beyond Token Change: Breaking The Cycle of Oppression in Institutions.* Fernwood Publishing

Branden, Nathaniel. 1994. *The Six Pillars of Self-Esteem*. Bantam Books.

Covey, Stephen. 2004. *The 7 Habits of Highly Effective People*. Free Press

Flaherty, James. 2005. *Coaching Evoking Excellence in Others. Third Edition*. Elsevier Butterworth-Heinemann.

Gilmore, S. and Fraleigh, P. 1993. *Communication at Work. & Style Profile Assessment.*

Hargrove, Robert. 2003. *Masterful Coaching*. Jossey Bass.

Humphrey, Holley. *Empathic Listening.* www.empathymagic.com.

John, Whitmore. 2004. *Coaching for Performance: Growing People, Performance and Purpose. Third Edition*. Nicholas Brealey Publishing.

Joyce, Stephen. 2007. *Teaching an Anthill to Fetch*. Mighty Small Books.

Lipsky, R.L. and Seeber D. F. 2003. *Emerging Systems for Managing Workplace Conflicts*. Jossey Bass.

Lopes, T. and Thomas, B. 2006. *Dancing on Live Embers: Challenging Racism in Organizations.* Fernwood Press.

Maxwell. John C.. 1998. *The 21 Irrefutable Laws of Leadership*. Thomas Nelson Publisher.

Odidison, Joyce. 2004. *Getting Ready for Mediation: A Pre-Mediation Concept.* Conflict Resolution Publishing.

Pollard. L, 2000. *Embracing Diversity: How to Understand and Reach People of All Cultures*. Review and Herald Publishing.

Redman, Warren. 2007. The 9 Steps to Emotional Fitness. Merlin Star Press

Senge, Peter M. 1990. *The Fifth Discipline The Art & Practice of The Learning Organization*. Doubleday Dell Publishing Group Inc.

Appendix A

If you begin the day with love in your heart, peace in your nerves, and truth in your mind, you not only benefit by their presence but also bring them to others, to your family and friends, and to all those whose destiny draws across your path that day.

-Unknown

Personal Feedback Questionnaire

Please carefully select the individuals whom you will be asking for feedback, to ensure you receive accurate information.

1. What do you think are my strengths?

    _____

    _____

    _____

    _____

2. What do you think is unique or special about me?

    _____

    _____

    _____

    _____

3. What do you think are my potentials or possibilities?

    _____

    _____

    _____

    _____

4. What do you think is my personality type or personal style?

    _____

    _____

    _____

    _____

5. What do you think are my excesses or areas for improvement?

_____

_____

_____

_____

6. What personal advice do you have for me?

_____

_____

_____

_____

7. What unrealized potentials do you think I may have?

_____

_____

_____

_____

8. What career or personal possibilities do you think I need to embrace or develop?

_____

_____

_____

_____

9. What environments do you think I work best in?

_____

_____

_____

_____

10. What do you think are my personal distractions?

_____

_____

_____

_____

11. What kinds of environments do you think I should personally or professionally avoid?

_____

_____

_____

_____

12. What do you think are my blind spots?

_____

_____

_____

_____

13. How do others speak of me?

_____

_____

_____

_____

14. What kinds of behaviours or actions do you expect from me?

_____

_____

_____

_____

15. Do you have any comments or suggestions not yet expressed above that you think may be beneficial for improving my Interpersonal Wellness?

_____

_____

_____

_____

_____

_____

_____

_____

_____

_____

_____

_____

_____

_____

_____

_____

_____

_____

_____

Thank you for taking the time to assist me in my Interpersonal Wellness development. I appreciate your interest in me.

Index

Interpersonal Wellness System

Book Order Form

Name: _____

Company: _____

Address: _____

City/Province: _____

Tel: _____ Fax: _____

E-Mail: _____

Cost of Book each: $24.95

Plus 5% GST

Please add $6.00 for shipping and handling costs in Canada, and $8.50 for orders outside Canada.

Total # of books ____

Order by fax, phone or e-mail: admin@interpersonalwellness.com

Make checks payable to Interpersonal Wellness Services Inc.

Method of Payment   Credit Card #

__ Check

                                _____

__ Bill Me   Expiry Date _____

__ Visa

__ Master Card   Signature

                                _____

Life Coaching Centre, IWS Inc
13 – 875 Gateway Rd. Winnipeg, MB R2K 4K6
Phone: 204 668-5283
Fax: 204 667-8845
Email: admin@interpersonalwellness.com

www.ingramcontent.com/pod-product-compliance
Lightning Source LLC
Chambersburg PA
CBHW060800270326
41926CB00002B/39